EXTRA
INNINGS

www.mascotbooks.com

*Extra Innings: Fred Claire's Journey to City of Hope
and Finding a World Championship Team*

Photographs courtesy of:
Bonnie Burrow
City of Hope
Fred Claire Collection
Jon Edwards
Richard Kee

For more information, please contact:
Mascot Books
620 Herndon Parkway #320
Herndon, VA 20170
info@mascotbooks.com

Library of Congress Control Number: 2020905560

CPSIA Code: PRFRE0420A
ISBN-13: 978-1-64543-083-4

Printed in Canada

For Fred and Sheryl Claire, and all the heroes at City of Hope—
humanity at its best.

EXTRA INNINGS

Fred Claire's Journey to City of Hope
and Finding a World Championship Team

Tim Madigan

Foreword by Bill Plaschke

Los Angeles Times

CONTENTS

FOREWORD *by Bill Plaschke* i

1 "FRED WAS THE PERFECT GUY" 1

2 SOMETHING IN THE AIR 17

3 A NASTY CANCER................................ 29

4 HISTORY IN THE MAKING 43

5 A DIFFERENT BALLGAME NOW 59

6 MAKINGS OF A MIRACLE....................... 69

7 DESTINY INTERVENES 83

8 HOW DO YOU EXPLAIN THAT?................. 99

9 FAMILY IS FAMILY.............................. 117

10 A VERY GOOD YEAR 141

11 STRAIGHT OUT OF HOLLYWOOD..............159

12 HOW WE HANDLE THE CHALLENGES 177

ACKNOWLEDGMENTS 199

FOREWORD

Bill Plaschke

Fred Claire is a fighter.

You might not know that to look at him—he's so distinguished and dignified and darned polite—but believe me, when he spots an unfairness or injustice, the man will come out swinging.

I know, because I've seen it. To be more exact, I've heard it.

It was the summer of 1990. I was the Dodgers' beat writer for the *Los Angeles Times*, and I was standing outside the closed door of Tom Lasorda's office in the bowels of Dodger Stadium. Inside the manager's room, one of the toughest players in Dodger history—the great Kirk Gibson—was staring down the kindly general manager, Fred Claire, trying to force Claire to trade him. Gibson thought he could push Claire around like he once pushed that Dennis Eckersley slider into the right-field pavilion for the most famous home run in Dodgers history. Gibson was wrong, and standing with my ear against that closed door, I could hear exactly how wrong.

"You're not doing your job. You need to trade me!" Gibson shouted.

"You're not going to tell me how to do my job!" Claire shouted back.

I heard shuffling and cursing and more shuffling.

"Have you ever seen a big bear in the woods?" Gibson shouted.

"No, do you know of any?" Claire responded.

There was more shuffling, more cursing, and I could have sworn I heard a punch thrown. I slowly backed away from the door, and moments later Gibson and Claire both stormed out and stalked away in different directions. Inside the office, Lasorda was still sitting at his desk, looking pale, as if he just witnessed something from a different world.

"Tommy, Tommy, did Gibby punch him?" I breathlessly asked.

"No, no, no, it was the other way around," said Lasorda. "Fred was going to punch Gibby!"

Soon there were clubhouse whispers about how Claire had actually taken off his sunglasses in preparation for battle with the legendary slugger and former football star.

"That's a bad man," said several players in admiration.

That, it turns out, is the real Fred Claire. Don't mistake his kindness for weakness. Don't think his brilliance prevents him from brawling. He cannot be bullied; he will not be intimidated.

When Claire took over the Dodgers' baseball operations in the wake of the Al Campanis scandal in the spring of 1987, he was dogged by the misconception that, as a former sportswriter, he was completely out of his league. He boldly fought back to make arguably the greatest set of personnel moves in Dodger history in building a 1988 World Series championship team whose accomplishments remain unmatched thirty-two years later.

Then, in 2015, he stared down another opponent: a deadly form of skin cancer that eventually moved into his jaw. Just as in his early days running the Dodgers, he wasn't given much of a chance to survive. But backed by the best corner men in the business at City of Hope National Medical Center in Duarte, California, he once again knocked out his nemesis.

In *Extra Innings*, Tim Madigan deftly chronicles both of Claire's winning fights, from his bold first Dodger signing of Mickey Hatcher to the recent inspiration he draws from City of Hope oncologist Dr. Erminia Massarelli. I am honored to write this foreword, not only because of my admiration for Claire, but also because of my appreciation for the special way this story is told. This is far more than a baseball book, it's a humanity book, and its pages abound with different heroes from different worlds, from Orel Hershiser and Mike Scioscia to City of Hope surgeon Dr. Thomas Gernon and patient navigator Lupe Santana.

I was lucky enough to cover the honorable Claire during his successful twelve-year regime as Dodger general manager. He was the most honest and integrity-driven sports executive I've ever met, yet I am more awed by his battle with cancer and insistence that the City of Hope be celebrated in the same manner as his champion Dodger team.

There are stories here not only about Gibson's famous home run, but also about the amazing Dr. Stephen Forman, a researcher and clinician whose leadership turned the medical center into one of the top stem-cell transplant facilities in the world. There is the story not only of Claire's deft handling of the Jay Howell pine tar scandal during that championship postseason of 1988 but also the compelling story behind City of Hope's researchers discovering the synthetic insulin that is commonly used by diabetics.

From Dodgertown to Duarte, these pages take us on an inspirational journey of perseverance, hope and, ultimately, triumph. For me, it is highlighted by the moment Claire had a crazy fundraising idea while sitting in an infusion room under-going cancer therapy. Even as he was clinging to life, he wanted to give life: "I said to myself, 'What is it that I can do to help? I'm getting all the help. What is it that I can do?'"

The results were two wildly successful consecutive celebrity golf tournaments that raised money for the medical center . . . two tournaments that Claire managed while undergoing chemotherapy.

"He would not buckle an inch . . . he met it head on," said the great Vin Scully of Claire's cancer battle. Scully could have also been talking about his baseball battle. The two fights are splendidly chronicled here in a story of a life too outsized for normal parameters, a life indeed worthy of extra innings.

1

"FRED WAS THE PERFECT GUY"

April 6, 1987

Al Campanis seemed a fitting guest for the ABC News program *Nightline*, which on that day in April was marking the fortieth anniversary of Jackie Robinson's Major League debut. Campanis had been a protégé of the legendary Brooklyn Dodgers executive Branch Rickey, the man who had helped shatter baseball's color barrier by promoting Robinson from the minors. Campanis moved with the team to Los Angeles in 1958 and had worked for the Dodgers in various administrative capacities ever since.

But to *Nightline* host Ted Koppel, Campanis' most important link to the Robinson fortieth anniversary story was personal.

"In 1946, he [Campanis] was a shortstop and teammate of

Jackie Robinson on a Brooklyn Dodgers farm team, the beginning of a close friendship that was to last until Robinson's death in 1972," Koppel said that night in introducing the man who was then the Dodgers' general manager and a team vice president.

Campanis was interviewed via satellite from the floor of the Houston Astrodome, where the Dodgers had just opened the season. Koppel immediately made clear that this would be no nostalgic puff piece, asking Campanis why, four decades after Robinson's watershed achievement, there were no black managers, general managers, or owners in Major League Baseball.

"The only thing I can say is that you have to pay your dues when you become a manager," Campanis said, implying that African Americans weren't willing to.

"You know in your heart of hearts that's a lot of baloney," Koppel said. "There are a lot of black players, a lot of great black baseball men, who would dearly love to be in managerial positions, and I guess what I'm really asking you is to peel it away a little bit. Just tell me, why do you think it is? Is there still that much prejudice in baseball today?"

"No, I don't believe it's prejudice," Campanis replied. "I truly believe they may not have some of the necessities to be, let's say, a field manager or perhaps a general manager."

"Do you really believe that?" an incredulous Koppel said. "That really sounds like garbage . . . I'm flabbergasted."

Later that night at the team hotel, Campanis ran into his old friend, the legendary Dodger broadcaster, Vin Scully.

"I think I screwed up," Campanis said.

"I'm sure it will be fine," Scully said, not knowing what had transpired during the interview. "Let's go have a bite to eat."

A shaken Campanis went to his room instead. Meanwhile,

reporters and editors were scrambling in newspaper sports departments across the nation.

The next morning in his Southern California home, Fred Claire was shocked when he opened his copy of the *Los Angeles Times*. He had been unaware of Campanis' *Nightline* appearance and was in disbelief while reading the story. Claire, himself a team vice president who had been part of the Dodger organization for eighteen years, considered Campanis a close friend.

"I couldn't believe what I was reading," Claire wrote in his 2004 autobiography, *My 30 Years in Dodger Blue*.

In Houston the next day, Campanis and team owner and president Peter O'Malley tried to calm a gathering firestorm with formal apologies. O'Malley insisted that his longtime general manager would not be fired, hoping that the tempest would blow over. But denunciations continued to pour in from across the nation, including one from Hall of Famer Hank Aaron, who said Campanis should "apologize to every single black person in America." Picketers converged on Dodger Stadium, where the team would soon hold its home opener. Campanis would have to go.

"The comments Al made Monday night . . . were so far removed and so distant from what I believe and what the organization believes that it was impossible for Al to continue the responsibilities that he's had with us," O'Malley said.

But who would take his place?

"Let's assume the *Nightline* thing had never happened," O'Malley said in an interview more than three decades later. "If Al had said, 'Hey Peter, I'm going to retire in another year,' no problem. Then we start a world search. But we didn't have that luxury. We didn't have time. It was opening day, and we needed someone quick."

Just before boarding his flight home from Texas, O'Malley made a telephone call.

"I had never heard Peter so down," Fred Claire wrote in his memoir. "His voice sounded as though he was calling from the bottom of a barrel. 'Fred,' he said, 'you have to take this job.'"

•◆•

The announcement of Campanis' successor raised eyebrows across baseball. For one thing, Fred Claire's name was likely to be unfamiliar to anyone not part of the local media or the Dodger organization. He was a trim, silver-haired man of fifty-one, who began his professional career as a sportswriter. Claire had been working the Dodger beat for a Long Beach newspaper at the time he joined the team's publicity department in 1969.

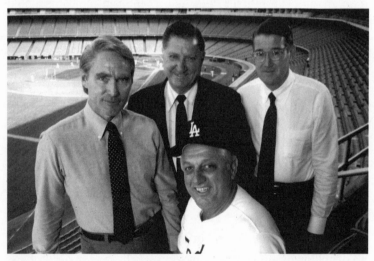

The leaders of the Dodgers during a long run with winning teams and record attendance were Fred, Al Campanis, Peter O'Malley, and Tommy Lasorda.

With the Dodgers, Claire was soon invited into the deliberations of the organization's top echelons. He became known for his ingenuity and tireless work ethic, but also integrity, humility, and quiet decency.

"Fred never lied to me. Never. Not once," Bill Plaschke, the longtime sports columnist of the *Los Angeles Times,* recalled in a 2019 interview. "He's the only person in that sort of position that I can say that about in all my years covering baseball. Their job is to lie to gain a competitive advantage. But Fred never did. If he couldn't tell you the truth, he wouldn't tell you anything at all. When Fred said, 'no comment,' you could almost take that to the bank as a 'yes.' I called him day and night, and he always took my calls, and he always answered my questions.

"He was like the small-town guy from Ohio that goes on to become president and governs with those same small-town values, integrity, and humility," Plaschke continued. "We used to think that Fred was boring, that Fred never said anything, but in saying so little he said so much."

In the mid-1970s, San Francisco Giants marketing director Pat Gallagher sought to boost ticket sales by fanning the flames of a historic baseball rivalry. "Hating the Dodgers" was the slogan he used to promote an upcoming series between the two teams.

Gallagher got a call from Los Angeles.

"Pat, 'hate' is too strong a word to be used carelessly to try to stir up emotion," Fred Claire told him. "We ought to be better than that. The objective isn't to promote violence. We don't really hate each other. We compete hard and try to beat each other on the field of play, but we always respect and help one another off the field. Find a different word for your ads."

Decades later, Gallagher recalled the conversation in a letter to Claire.

"I was stunned and embarrassed to be called out by one of the most respected people in the game," Gallagher wrote. "I never forgot your advice and appreciated it more than you'll ever know."

Five years after joining the Dodgers organization, Claire was promoted to the position of vice president for marketing. He was the one who coined the phrase Dodger Blue, which would soon rival the Yankees' pinstripes and the Dallas Cowboys' star among the most iconic brands in professional sports.

On April 25, 1976, Claire played a central role in one of the most memorable moments in Dodger history. In that afternoon's game at Dodger Stadium against the Cubs, two men stole onto the outfield grass, spread out an American flag, doused it with lighter fluid, and prepared to set it on fire. At the last second, Cubs outfielder Rick Monday dashed in and snatched the flag away.

Jeff Fellenzer, a young intern, was running the Dodger message board that day. Claire, then the team's director of marketing, was sitting a few feet away and overseeing press box operations.

"When this was all happening, it was hard to understand what was going on," Fellenzer recalled in a 2019 interview. "But Fred turned to me and said, 'Jeff, type these words. Rick Monday, dot, dot, dot . . . You made a great play . . . ' You talk about thinking quick on your feet. That was Fred's take on what had happened."

Within seconds, the crowd rose and spontaneously began to sing God Bless America. Claire's phone rang in the press box. It was team owner Walter O'Malley.

"Fred, this will go down as one of the greatest moments in Dodger Stadium history," O'Malley said.

By that fateful spring of 1987, Claire's title was executive vice president. In the team hierarchy, he was just below Peter O'Malley, who had succeeded his father as Dodger owner.

But Claire had never played an inning of professional baseball.

"He had been a sportswriter, for crying out loud," *Los Angeles Times* columnist Jim Murray wrote in 1987. "His specialty was marketing and promotion."

There were whispers that more experienced general managers on other teams would trade him blind.

"Campanis had his faults, but he knew the game," a veteran Dodger player told a reporter at the time. "I have no idea what to expect now."

To greatly compound matters, the team was in shambles. Long gone were the days of legendary stars like Sandy Koufax and Don Drysdale, Steve Garvey, Ron Cey, and Davey Lopes. There were fewer postseason appearances, and the most recent World Series title had been in 1981.

"Everywhere you looked, the Dodgers were in disarray," Murray wrote. "Like the French army, it wasn't even a retreat, it was a rout. The starting pitching was terrible, the relief pitching nonexistent. Third basemen were playing first, outfielders were playing third, the lineup consisted almost wholly of utility players, triple-A players, or guys who long since should have gone home to sell real estate or insurance."

Hence the titters and whispers among outsiders. But there were many things about Fred Claire they would not know. One was the nature of his relationship with O'Malley, with whom he shared a bond based on trust and mutual respect.

"Peter was a very thoughtful guy, and he had a legacy to protect—the legacy of the Dodger organization, the family-owned Dodgers," said Peter Bavasi, a longtime Major League Baseball executive. He is also the son of Buzzie Bavasi, another club legend and a predecessor of Campanis as the Dodgers' general manager. "He wasn't going to put that at risk by hiring someone who wasn't going to do the right things, say the right things, build the right sort of club. And he was close to Fred. He liked Fred. I remember at meetings when the two of them were together, you could tell they were very close by the way they chatted with one another, the way they spoke to one another, their gestures toward one another. It was a very special relationship."

Nor would outsiders know how Claire had been preparing for this moment for nearly two decades, though not in a traditional way. Sportswriters joked that one of their own was now running the team, but from the beginning of his time with the Dodgers, Claire had put his journalistic skills to good use, working with the doggedness and curiosity of an investigative reporter. He learned the organization from top to bottom and got to know every person in it, from the team president to the players, from the clubhouse attendants to the network of talent scouts in whom the Dodgers took great pride.

He had also sat in on hundreds of meetings over the years, listening as Campanis and baseball men like managers Walter Alston and Tommy Lasorda, and Bill Schweppe, head of minor league operations, discussed the intricacies of team construction and talent evaluation.

"That talk [of a lack of baseball background] doesn't bother me, because I'll ultimately be judged in terms of performance," Claire told a reporter. "I'm certainly not uncomfortable with it. There were hundreds of days when I'd have lunch with Walter and Peter O'Malley, Bill [Schweppe] and Al. I'd spend hours talking about the game and the business of baseball. I learned a great deal from all of them. It was like getting a master's degree in baseball."

Finally, Claire was not only knowledgeable, he was also fiercely competitive, as anyone who saw him on the tennis court or shared a jogging trail could attest. And he seemed utterly undaunted by the challenge thrust upon him; witness his terms when O'Malley asked him to take the job:

"Peter, I will accept the job, but under one condition," Claire said on the day of the team's home opener.

"What is that?"

"I want to have total and complete responsibility [for baseball operations]," Claire said.

The reason? He wanted the world to know who would be accountable if things with the team went further south.

"It's a very difficult job. It's a job that gets a lot of second guessing," Claire told an interviewer years later. "I thought it was very important for all of the members of the Dodger organization—and, just as importantly, for the fans—to understand who was making the decisions, who was in charge. Not to say, 'Look how much authority I have,' but if I was a customer, I think I would like to know. You needed to have that mindset of accepting the responsibility and accountability and not blaming others."

In the end, for all the whispers, it turned out that Fred Claire was the perfect person for such a difficult moment.

"It was terrible—an incredibly volatile time like no other

in the history of the Dodgers," said Plaschke, the *Los Angeles Times* writer. "It was a disaster. Peter O'Malley needed someone to calm the waters, and Fred was the perfect guy. He was an incredibly standup person. He was smart, and he was fearless. He was stepping into one of the most visible, pressurized positions in all of sports, and he didn't flinch. Fred became the face and voice of the Dodgers, and it was a calm and decent voice. He spoke with a quiet voice, a dignified voice."

But Claire knew there were no guarantees after the waters had been calmed.

"I'll do it until he says don't do it anymore," he told a reporter early on, speaking of O'Malley. "Peter is the president of this company. If he says there is a better man for this job, fine."

Only one thing was certain.

"I knew I was going to do this job to the best of my ability every day," Claire said. "When I was appointed, Peter was asked, 'How long does Fred have the job?' The answer, I believe, was, 'He has it for today.' And that's all we really have. In our jobs and in our lives. All that we really have is today, so I think it is imperative for all of us to do the best we can today."

Yet from the outset, Claire also made it clear he was not content to be a seat warmer. In his second day as general manager, he signed veteran Mickey Hatcher, a player known for his passion for the game and his infectious positive attitude, and released Jerry Reuss, a popular veteran pitcher and one of the team's highest paid players.

"The league expected Claire's administration to be one of 'don't make waves and thus don't make mistakes,'" Murray wrote in the *Times*. "They thought he would just try to keep the ship afloat till management could hire a real general manager, one wise in the ways and chicanery of baseball's front offices.

"To the complete surprise of everyone, Claire began making noises like a guy who intends to attack. He didn't feel as if they had handed him a disaster; they had given him an opportunity. He rolled up his sleeves and went to work . . . Baseball knew that Fred Claire didn't see himself as anybody's stopgap."

His tenure, as it turned out, would stretch on for more than a decade, making him one of the longest serving general managers of his time. Within two years of his hiring, Claire had helped orchestrate a storybook season that ended with the Dodgers shocking a heavily favored Oakland team and winning the 1988 World Series. Thirty-one years later, frustrated Dodger fans were still awaiting another title.

Given all that, no one could have foreseen that Fred Claire's greatest challenge, and perhaps his greatest achievements, would come long after he left the game.

•◆•

Beginning in 2015, a devastating form of skin cancer would be his foe in a battle that Fred Claire, soon to be eighty years old, took on with his trademark fortitude. He would need every bit of it. With his wife, Sheryl, at his side, he would be tested as never before, then tested again, and again. But through years of physical pain and grueling emotional challenges, he refused to give in to despair, stubbornly choosing to focus on the good.

The bonds of his thirty-year marriage grew even stronger, as did his relationship with his children. Fred came to have an even deeper appreciation for the opportunities he had been given, the experiences he had enjoyed, friendships he had formed both in and out of baseball, and the fragility and preciousness of life.

He became even more acutely aware of the fact that cancer was no respecter of the game. Friends like slugger Don Baylor and general manager Kevin Towers were both taken by the disease too soon. He met and befriended a high school baseball coach named Tom Quinley, who would also lose his battle to lung cancer. One day on a high school playing field, Claire addressed Quinley's players and met one of them, a gutsy pitcher and leukemia survivor named Jaylon Fong. Fong had pitched and won the season opener on the day the team retired Quinley's number.

Throughout, Fred would not focus only on his own healing.

"My good fortune drives me forward," he said in the spring of 2019. "I've never felt more strongly about anything. We have an opportunity to contribute and we can contribute more. When you go through cancer, I guess the right word is empathy: you feel empathy for others. You feel it in your heart and in your soul. You want to help."

With his own survival hardly guaranteed, Fred marshalled what remained of his energies and focused them outward. His primary mission became shining a light on City of Hope National Medical Center in a Los Angeles suburb or, more specifically, on the doctors, nurses, researchers, administrators, patient advocates, and volunteers there who joined him and his wife in the fight for healing.

The new mission was inspired in part by a conversation with television's Tom Brokaw, who had undertaken his own recent fight with the blood cancer multiple myeloma.

"Tom had worked in Los Angeles and had been on the board of Mayo Clinic," Fred said. "But when we were talking about my situation, he said, 'I'm sure it's a fine place, but I don't know about City of Hope.' That made me start to wonder whether the world really knew what a gift it had here."

Sitting in the shadow of the San Gabriel Mountains, City of Hope was one of the great stories in American medicine; though, Fred Claire felt it was largely untold. From the moment they stepped on campus, he and Sheryl were struck by the compassion and humility of everyone they met, from CEO Robert Stone to oncologist Dr. Erminia Massarelli, and from surgeon Thomas Gernon to patient navigator Lupe Santana. That humanity, it turned out, had been baked into the DNA of the century-old institution from the start.

"What I have consistently found in my twenty-three years here is a focus on paying it forward, a dedication to truly helping others," Stone, the CEO, said in the spring of 2019. "Egos have to be checked at the door. People who come with huge egos, they don't last very long here. While we may have had some over the years, you have to make yourself smaller than the greater good to last."

Which wouldn't matter greatly if not for the other components of the institution's magic. For decades, City of Hope has been a leader in the treatment of diabetes and helped pioneer bone marrow and stem cell transplantation. By the time Fred arrived to take up his fight, the center had leapfrogged to the forefront of the revolution in cancer research and treatment. There are few other places in the world where, for example, cancer researchers can explore potential cures on laboratory benches just a few hundred yards from the bedsides of patients who would ultimately benefit. City of Hope has developed a system to get patients registered for potentially life-saving clinical trials more quickly and efficiently than almost anywhere else. As part of a dramatic expansion, scores of the world's top researchers and clinicians have found their way to the City of Hope campus in recent years.

"I think we've become the premiere cancer program on the planet, and it's a result of the talent that's come here and the capacity of City of Hope to advance discoveries to patients on campus," Dr. Steven Rosen, M.D., the institution's provost and chief scientific officer, said in a 2019 interview.

That was the story Fred Claire wanted to tell the world. It was while sitting in an infusion room undergoing chemotherapy that he conceived of the first of two wildly successful celebrity golf tournaments that raised hundreds of thousands of dollars and generated waves of local publicity for City of Hope.

"I looked at him and I said, 'Fred, are you crazy?'" Sheryl remembered. "You must be the only guy in chemo with a 20 percent chance of survival planning a golf tournament.'"

On New Year's Day in 2018, Fred joined nine other patients to ride on the City of Hope float in the Rose Parade. He threw out the first pitch at Dodger Stadium and was the topic of several news stories in which City of Hope was prominently mentioned. He joined the lecture circuit with the same message.

"I want the world to know how I feel about these people," he said. "I couldn't invent this. Nothing is contrived. Everything is real. This is the greatest team I've ever been involved with. I've known great players and great teams. I've never had the opportunity to be involved in anything like this."

Once again, Fred Claire would be the perfect person for a difficult moment.

"He would not buckle an inch," broadcaster Vin Scully said in 2019 of his longtime friend. "He met it head on. And with all the baseball things behind him, what he's done with the cancer, living through all the mental and physical pain, that's his greatest accomplishment. He couldn't top that in baseball if he tried.

"It was almost as if God said, 'You're not working with the Dodgers, but you can be inspirational to millions of people. That's your job now.' Those who know about him, who come in contact with him, who hear about what he's on Earth for now, realize he has been given a job that is a heck of a lot more important and bigger in stature than being the general manager of a baseball team."

2

SOMETHING IN THE AIR

City of Hope sprawls over more than a hundred acres in Duarte, about thirty miles northeast of downtown Los Angeles. On any typical day, clinicians, researchers, administrators, nurses, volunteers, support staff, and patients hurry back and forth between the medical center's earth-toned buildings; occasionally, though, they pause for a few restorative minutes in places of natural beauty and quiet.

One is the Japanese Garden—featuring arrays of flowers, a wooden bridge, a waterfall, and a pond stocked with colorful koi—tucked into the campus between a science building and the visitor center. Another is the International Garden of Meditation, a rose garden along the northern border of the campus. There you also find a City of Hope touchstone. It is the Golter Gate, named for an early leader of the institution, Samuel H. Golter. The gate is made of gold-plated wrought iron and bears the words of Golter's motto:

"There is no profit in curing the body if, in the process, we destroy the soul."

Golter had come to City of Hope in 1926, thirteen years after residents of a Jewish neighborhood in Southern California watched a homeless young victim of tuberculosis collapse and die on the street.

The disease from which he suffered was one of the world's great scourges of the time, known as "consumption" because it consumed the body, or the "white plague." Invariably fatal, tuberculosis was particularly devastating to immigrant populations toiling in East Coast sweatshops. Most hospitals refused to admit tuberculosis victims because of the contagious nature of the disease.

"Stricken members of devoted families were often forced, or even chose to leave their homes in the hope of preventing the spread of infection to those who had yet escaped the scourge," Golter wrote in his memoir, *The City of Hope*. "The outcasts were herded into derelict or dilapidated buildings, which had been thrown open to them along the crowded eastern seaboard."

Sunshine and a dry climate were thought to be curative, hence the thousands of tuberculosis sufferers and their families who made their way to the West Coast in the early part of the twentieth century. After witnessing the agonizing death of the young tuberculosis victim, residents of the Jewish neighborhood in Southern California collected $136.05 for a down payment on a few acres in Duarte.

"It was 1913 that the two tents were set up—one for patients, the other for a nurse," Golter wrote. "Nothing could be done medically to save the lives of the patients, but they were saved the indignity of dying on the streets. Such were the humble and humanitarian beginnings of the City of Hope."

By the time of Golter's arrival, the place consisted of about ten wood-frame cottages and a few stucco buildings. But it was something less tangible about the place that inspired his lifelong commitment.

"I became aware of an unaccountable 'something' in the air," Golter wrote. "Before too long I had identified the mysterious element as a spirit of kindness and goodwill which was manifested toward the patients to a degree that was unprecedented in my experience . . . the founders and supporters of the sanatorium were determined to preserve the dignity of suffering people."

Under Golter's leadership, and with the financial help of members of the movie industry and grassroots contributors, the campus eventually expanded to include a hospital and research facility.

"In recognition of the opportunity given me to maintain the dignity of those who had fallen by the wayside," Golter wrote, "I coined the slogan which became our watchword."

In the years after World War II, antibiotics had largely eradicated tuberculosis and, as a result, the original mission of City of Hope had become mercifully obsolete. But Golter believed that the institution's founding spirit could be brought to bear against other devastating afflictions. Its purpose would come to include research into and treatment of cancer, diabetes, and heart disease.

"When I finally had the medical center clearly blueprinted in my mind, I felt more than ever that in enlarging the scope of our services we could satisfy both of the entities of man—the spiritual as well as the physical," he wrote. "The thought of creating a City of Hope Medical Center was rarely out of my mind. I convinced myself that we, the people of the City of Hope, could and would create the first medical center on the American scene to have the unique objective of adding 'life to years' as well as 'years to life.'"

A City of Hope research institute was formally established in 1952. That same year, Golter was succeeded as CEO by a New York-trained lawyer named Ben Horowitz, who combined the same commitment to humanitarianism with a genius for fundraising. During his tenure, Horowitz expanded the City of Hope annual budget. It went from $600,000 when he started to $100 million by his retirement in 1985.

A young researcher named Susumu Ohno arrived in Duarte the same year as Horowitz, though somewhat less auspiciously. Ohno was a research associate with a doctorate in veterinary medicine, but he would eventually be credited with groundbreaking discoveries in the fields of genetics, epigenetics, and molecular evolution that would have profound implications in the fight against disease. Among those to take notice was Arthur Riggs, a young researcher at the Salk Institute just south of Los Angeles.

"I was interested in how genes were regulated and how they were turned on and off," Riggs remembered in 2019. "I started looking for a place where I could have my own laboratory and do my own research. And I learned that at the City of Hope there was a brilliant scientist, Dr. Ohno. I was lucky enough for him to offer me a position in his department. That was one of the best decisions of my career, to come to the City of Hope."

When he arrived in 1969, Riggs found a small but brilliant group of researchers, as well as physician/scientists like Dr. Ernest Beutler, a German-born hematologist whose work at

City of Hope included helping to pioneer bone marrow transplantation. Riggs was also struck by the culture of care that had endured from City of Hope's early days.

"The goal was to help humanity by alleviating or curing all of the catastrophic diseases," Riggs said. "Our goal was to help people. Our goal was to cure disease, and I was very much influenced by and adopted the culture.

"It was very collaborative," he said. "Sure, we try to be successful for ourselves, but really, we're trying to help others."

To that end, Riggs and his City of Hope colleagues succeeded in a historic way. In January 1979, the National Academy of Science published the findings of Riggs and researcher Keiichi Itakura—an article that detailed one of the most significant medical breakthroughs of the twentieth century.

Until that time, insulin that was needed to manage the symptoms of diabetes was harvested from the pancreases of cows. Because it was an animal product, some diabetes patients suffered allergic reactions. What's more, eight thousand animal organs were needed to produce one pound of insulin, and the drug was prohibitively expensive as a result.

Riggs and others worked in the laboratory for much of the 1970s to come up with an alternative. Using biotechnology, they created a new gene that when combined with bacteria caused the bacteria to produce insulin. The result was man-made, synthetic insulin, which was the first drug created by biotechnology ever approved by the U.S. Food and Drug Administration for human use.

Ironically, on the day of a momentous breakthrough, Riggs found himself in the same place as Fred Claire.

"On the afternoon our team was trying to see if insulin had

been made, we were huddled around an instrument that measured the production of the desired protein that led to insulin," he recalled. "The first day we got a positive signal, we thought we were all successful, so we all were quite excited about it. We shook hands and agreed that it looked good, that we probably had it. But then I had to leave because I had promised to take my son to a Dodger game.

"Dodger Stadium was an awesome environment. It's really beautiful. In this amazing setting, while the game was going on, I was thinking about all the possible implications of what we did and what came to be the biotechnology revolution. I don't remember very much about the game, but I do remember that's how I celebrated with my son."

By 1982, synthetic insulin that went by the brand name Humulin was available commercially. Nearly four decades later, it remains a standard of care drug for diabetes sufferers worldwide.

"I do feel good about it," Riggs said in the spring of 2019. "Our research has helped a lot of people, but I don't dwell on it. I'm orientated toward the future. It's not what I've done; it's what I'm trying to do now. I mostly think about the next disease we're going to cure and, of course, I want to cure diabetes. That's what I spend my time thinking about."

•◆•

In 1978, a young oncologist/researcher named Dr. Stephen Forman treated several leukemia patients at the medical center of the University of Southern California. All of them died.

"I wanted to be part of something that would change the

outcomes for those people," Forman said years later.

He found his opportunity in an unlikely place: a small medical center in the little-known suburb of Duarte. Despite its obscurity, City of Hope was one of only six facilities in the United States experimenting with the use of bone marrow and stem cell transplantation to treat blood cancers.

It was a risky, radical procedure: destroying a patient's diseased bone marrow with high doses of chemotherapy, then reintroducing healthy stem cells that would find their way back into the bone marrow and begin to recreate healthy blood and immune systems.

"Basically, I came for a six- to eight-week rotation, and I decided I wasn't going back to USC except to get my stuff," Forman said in 2019. "It was exciting. We were doing something that had never been done. In retrospect, I came to recognize how on the edge we were. I can't say we completely understood every detail of it, and so we were developing things and improving things almost with each patient."

But it was more than the cutting-edge science that inspired Forman to make his career in Duarte. At the time, City of Hope was the only one of the pioneering transplant programs not associated with a major university.

"We're not the University of City of Hope, we're City of Hope," he said. "We were also a relatively small place. I think there was more of an appetite for doing things that were new. We were people from different backgrounds, different ages, different countries. But I think we all knew what we were trying to do, which was to take this person who was going to die from a cancer and try to prevent that from happening. The way it was run then, and the way we run it now, is that any idea that's a good idea matters more than who came up with it.

"It gave me and the people with whom I worked an opportunity to try to make a change, not just for the patients we see at City of Hope, but maybe across the world if our dreams were realized."

Stem cell transplantation would revolutionize treatment of leukemia and other blood related cancers, such as multiple myeloma, curing many patients and greatly extending the lives of others. By 2019, City of Hope remained one of the top-rated stem cell transplant facilities in the world, having performed more than 15,000 of the procedures. An annual Celebration of Life event brings together more than 7,000 City of Hope transplant survivors.

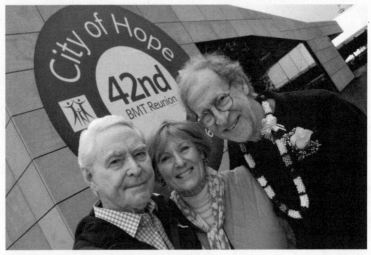

City of Hope invites bone marrow transplant recipients and their families to attend the annual Celebration of Life event. Fred and Sheryl attended the 42nd reunion and visited with Dr. Stephen Forman.

Over the decades, Forman came to be seen as the embodiment of the place where he worked. A thin, soft-spoken man with a close-cropped beard and graying hair often pulled into a stubby ponytail, he was both a cutting-edge researcher and a clinician who immersed himself in the lives of his patients.

"Research is done because I see the need to improve things and do things better. Taking care of people keeps it real," said Forman, who would also come to be a leader in City of Hope immunotherapy research, the new therapy that revolutionized cancer treatment. "Taking care of other human beings is a privilege. I get as much from them as I give to them."

He acknowledges the emotional and scientific challenges of a life practicing a form of medicine that is experimental and risky by nature. Yet to him and others at City of Hope, emotional detachment is never an option.

"But you have to conduct clinical trials in a way that the patient feels like they are the most valuable person in our lives," he said. "I hear it from patients in other places, the guinea pig concept. When you're on a clinical trial, everybody loves you; you're getting cared for. But if you go off the trial for whatever reason, because of toxicity or it's not working, suddenly they're not as interested in you anymore. That cannot be. Here we believe that if we grab your hand, we're not letting it go. We go where you go.

"We get asked this question all the time, 'What if it was your brother, your child, your mother, your buddy?'" Forman said. "What I've always said is, 'If she's sitting across from me, she is my wife, you are my brother. You are my friend.' So it's not as if we would take care of anybody any differently than we would our parent, our children, our siblings. That is, I believe, what accounts for our success."

In fact, the patients that Forman couldn't cure are often the ones he remembers most: "For every breakthrough that we have had, all of us can think about somebody that we knew or cared for or took care of here that, if we had known then what we know now, they'd be around, too. So, there is this urgency. The day isn't long enough. We get our work done because somebody is going to be knocking on our door tonight or tomorrow, and we want to be ready in a way that is better than it was yesterday. We can't be living in yesterday. People don't come here for that. They want tomorrow's therapy today."

•◆•

In 2017, with his plans for a benefit golf tournament taking shape, Fred Claire stepped out of an elevator on the floor of Forman's office. The first thing Fred saw was the framed jersey of his friend, Don Baylor, the baseball slugger, who had been diagnosed with multiple myeloma in 2003 and was a patient of Forman's until Baylor's death in August 2017.

That day, in their first meeting, it was quickly established that Fred and Forman shared a deep passion for baseball in general and the Dodgers in particular. Early in their conversation, Forman playfully asked Fred what the number forty-two meant to him. The former general manager chuckled because the answer was obvious.

"Well, that was and always will be Jackie Robinson's number," he said.

Claire had, in fact, met and had been with Robinson on several occasions over the years, the last being in Cincinnati in 1972 when Robinson threw out the honorary first ball before a World Series game. That day, Claire watched as the baseball legend embraced an old Brooklyn Dodger teammate, Pee Wee Reese, who Robinson could not see as Reese approached because of diabetes-related blindness. A few minutes later, Robinson told a national television audience, "I'd like to see a black manager. I'd like to see the day when there is a black man coaching third base." Robinson died nine days later.

In 2017, at a banquet following his first golf tournament to benefit City of Hope, Fred presented the Celebration of Life trophy to another baseball great: Rod Carew. It bore Robinson's words, "A life is not important except in the impact it has on other lives."

That was exactly what Fred wanted the spirit of his tournament to represent. Robinson had articulated what Fred had witnessed on every trip to City of Hope, where every patient was treated not only with the best medical care that science had to offer but also with a profound compassion.

During their first meeting, Forman told Fred that he was also a great admirer of Robinson. But when asking his question, he had something else in mind. The next year, he told Fred, would be the forty-second anniversary of the first stem cell transplant at City of Hope, and he invited Fred and his wife to attend the next reunion of survivors.

For Fred, he wasn't just meeting a doctor: "This was a connection from the soul. And when you meet him [Forman], there is a power and a grace about him because of what he does. You can't help but be touched by it, because that's just who he is."

Fred added, "We had felt this from so many other people at City of Hope by then, but it all comes from the top. Meeting Dr. Forman tied it all together. You realized these great and caring people were not isolated. They were part of a philosophy, a program and that always begins at the top. I had just met somebody who truly cares about other people. You could ask a hundred patients and I'm sure they would all feel that Dr. Forman isn't their doctor: he is their friend."

3

A NASTY CANCER

I t began with a spot on the left side of Fred's lower lip, one so small that even his wife, Sheryl, didn't notice it. The only worrisome thing about the spot was that it did not go away. In January 2015, after a biopsy, a dermatologist diagnosed it as squamous cell carcinoma, a potentially deadly form of skin cancer. Though the initial news was terrifying, the prognosis was hopeful after a surgery, known as a Mohs procedure, that took place on January 28. The cancer did not appear to have spread to surrounding tissue, and doctors were confident it had been completely removed. Fred and Sheryl resumed an active and happy life.

Fred's thirty-year career with the Dodgers had come to a painful and controversial end seventeen years before, when he was fired by new corporate owners who purchased the team from Peter O'Malley. Fred never took another full-time job in baseball but stayed connected with the game through a column and radio show, *GM Corner*, for MLB.com; as a consultant for several sports related companies; and by forming a baseball analytics company with a friend, Ari Kaplan.

Fred had also focused much of his energies in the post-baseball years on college teaching, lecturing in the first ever class in "sports business" at the prestigious Caltech (where Kaplan had been a student), and helping to launch sports business programs at the University of Southern California and Long Beach State. He served on the Rose Bowl's board of directors and helped organize the First Tee golf program in Pasadena to help introduce young people to the game he loved.

In 2011, Fred Claire's name returned to the headlines, thanks to a former Dodger batboy named Ben Hwang. That year, Dodger owner Frank McCourt had once again put the team up for sale. Soon after the news broke, Hwang contacted his old friend and mentor. Fred had first met Ben in 1984, the seventeen-year-old's first year as a Dodger batboy. After three years working in the dugout and clubhouse, Fred promoted him to the team's front office.

"I was so low on the totem pole that one of my jobs was picking people up at the airport, including Fred," Ben recalled in a 2019 interview. "Though our interactions were few, he was always so interested in what I was doing. When I would have thirty minutes alone in the car with him, he would always ask about my family, how things were going, and how the office was."

Fred later encouraged the young man to enroll at USC. Ben Hwang went on to obtain a doctorate in biology from Johns Hopkins University and founded a biotech company in the San Francisco Bay Area that grew rapidly.

On June 25, 2011, Fred received this message:

I must apologize for the radio silence for so long, but I hope you understand that life's daily activities have a certain way of making time go by without one's notice. However, I have been following the news regarding our beloved Dodgers and have read a few articles where you have been quoted. It reminded me to get in touch with you and let you know that the opportunities you gave me at Dodger Stadium so many years ago are the direct cause of so much good that has happened in my life. I can draw a direct link of all of the major events in my life back to those wonderful experiences with the Dodgers . . . thank you.

I know you must be busy, Mr. Claire, but I am going to be in the Los Angeles/San Diego area next week to attend to some business. I would love the chance to grab lunch or just meet face-to-face to catch up and say thanks for all you've done for me.

• ◆ •

But something else was also on Ben Hwang's mind: With Fred Claire's guidance, he believed he could pursue a childhood fantasy of owning the Dodgers. The former general manager didn't hesitate when the former batboy asked him to join the prospective ownership group. At Fred's urging, Ben also persuaded highly regarded former Major League Baseball executives Andy Dolich and Dick Freeman to join the effort.

"There was so much interest in buying the team. The odds of success were always stacked against us, but it was a fabulous ride, and I'm just so thankful that Fred came back into my life in that project," Ben said. "He was my partner in every sense of the word. And because of his career and his standing within the baseball community, he allowed my group to have much greater credibility. We really had a fundamental orientation to make this work and try to get the Dodgers back to where they really needed to be. Because of his involvement, we were able to articulate a vision that was really compelling."

While the two were at lunch one day, Ben was somewhat starstruck when Fred took a call from another friend who expressed interest in joining their team—Ernie Banks, the legendary Chicago Cub Hall of Famer.

Ben Hwang's group was a finalist in the Dodger sweepstakes, but eventually lost out to another group headed by basketball great Magic Johnson. As their prospective business partnership dissolved, a cherished friendship between Ben and Fred deepened.

"He was such a good role model for me that I couldn't help but develop a fondness for him," Ben said. "I would like to think that he is proud of our friendship and proud of my accomplishments because of the way he was able to impact me. He is just so committed to doing the right thing every day. He lives those virtues day in and day out, in private and in public. His value system doesn't change behind doors, or when you're having breakfast or lunch with him at Pie 'n Burger in Pasadena, or when he's at a World Series press conference in front of a hundred reporters. The modeling of that behavior, that's incredibly powerful."

•◆•

Fred's idyllic post-baseball life continued as he approached his eightieth birthday in 2015. He looked a decade younger, thanks to a busy lifestyle, a healthy diet, and regular exercise. He remained passionately engaged in college classrooms, offering to mentor any student who showed up at his Pasadena office. He maintained close relationships with dozens of former Dodger players, employees, and executives.

"There is not a Dodger from that time in the 1980s that Fred doesn't still know," said *Los Angeles Times* columnist Bill Plaschke. "And they all talk to Fred. They'll call and ask his advice about careers, baseball, families, business, ethics. Everyone just looks up to him."

Fred and his wife could also be seen traipsing across a golf course, always eschewing a cart to walk and tote their own bags. When it came, the cancer scare seemed only that, a scare—a sobering but brief diversion. Fred Claire resumed teaching in the winter of 2015 with a bandage on his lip. But as months passed, something didn't seem right. He could still feel a spot on his lip, but on several occasions, his doctor dismissed it as scar tissue from the surgery.

"My appointments basically consisted of you taking a picture of my lip and then moving on to the next patient," Fred said in a letter to that doctor in 2017. "With my mention of feeling a spot on my lip, there never was the suggestion of any type of exam to determine if there was something that might need to be addressed. What I didn't realize is what a potentially dangerous area the lip is related to the cancer cells."

Sheryl Claire also regretted not being a more forceful advocate for her husband. "I didn't go with Fred to those visits. Now, I would just say to the doctor, 'Why is this still evident? What is there?'" she said. "I would have also said, 'Why can't we have an MRI? Why can't we have a scan?' But I wasn't there, and we weren't aware enough. We put too much trust in him."

In his letter, Fred urged the doctor to be more open to additional exams and second opinions with patients in the future. The experience underscored advice Fred was given by Tom Brokaw.

"You have to be the captain of your own ship," Brokaw said. "Fred, never be afraid to get a second opinion."

By August 2016, it could no longer be denied. Something was very wrong. At first, Fred attributed the searing pain in his face, neck, and jaw to an infection from a recent tooth extraction. He would wake up with mild discomfort, but as the day progressed, so did the pain. There were times while driving home in the afternoon that the agony would cause him to scream: "It was so intolerable that in the evening, I would lay on the couch for one or two minutes, move to the bedroom for one or two minutes, move someplace else for one or two minutes. It was inescapable. It was the worst pain you could ever imagine, and the strongest pain medication didn't really help."

His doctor finally ordered scans of his jaw and neck. On Wednesday, September 21, 2016, Fred had just gotten behind the wheel of his car when his cell phone rang.

"You have squamous cell carcinoma in your jaw," the doctor said. "This is serious and must be addressed."

Two days after the doctor's referral, Fred and Sheryl made the short drive from their home in Pasadena to the City of Hope campus in Duarte, where they had been only once before to visit Fred's longtime secretary, Rosie Gutierrez, who later lost her battle with cancer. Now their minds raced as they walked from the parking lot hand in hand, passing the Spirit of Life statue and fountain to the main patient entrance.

After completing necessary paperwork, the Claires were shown into an exam waiting room. The experience there was familiar to all cancer patients and their loved ones: agonizing minutes waiting for a new doctor to walk through the door for the first time, often to deliver bad news. The experience seemed surreal, and Sheryl was terrified: "Never, ever in our wildest dreams did I think that this little spot he had on his lip, one that was removed, would end up causing him such horrific pain. I never would have dreamed it would end up being cancer in his jaw and other places and that we would be fighting for our lives."

Fred recalls looking across the exam room at his wife. "Sheryl was somewhat silent. I could clearly read the look on her face—very, very scared. I think my own reaction may have been very different at thirty or forty or fifty or even seventy. I realized how blessed I had been to have such good health over so many years. You've lived your life, and you realize how blessed you've been. I just knew that I now had a hell of a challenge in front of me."

As they sat there, the Claires were also deeply curious about the physician about to walk through the door, the person who would become as important to them as a family member. Of course, they had read up on Dr. Thomas J. Gernon, who was reputed to be one of the finest head and neck surgeons in the nation.

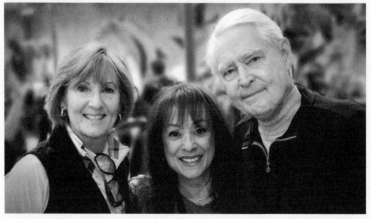

City of Hope patient navigator Lupe Santana was one of the first people Fred and Sheryl met at the medical center. "Navigators like Lupe are a part of the caring culture at City of Hope and play a key role in assisting patients," says Fred.

Gernon had come to City of Hope just a few months before as part of the wave of top clinicians and researchers recruited to Duarte in the last few years. He certainly had impressive credentials. The young physician had founded the head and neck oncology program at the University of Arizona Medical Center and developed one of the largest referral centers in Southern Arizona for patients with complex tumors in those parts of the body. His articles had appeared in prestigious medical journals, and he had lectured across the nation.

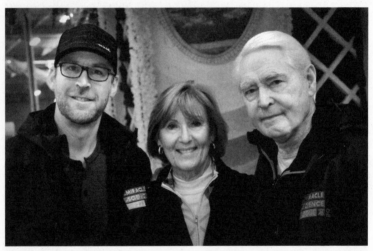

Dr. Thomas Gernon and Fred were on the City of Hope float in the Rose Parade in 2018. Dr. Gernon performed surgery on Fred in 2016 and 2019 in his battle against head and neck cancer.

There was finally a knock on the door, and a tall, thin man, about forty years old, stepped into the room. He wore casual clothes and carried a file. He extended his hand to Fred Claire.

"Pleased to meet you, Dr. Gernon," Fred said.

But this would not be the typical doctor-patient relationship.

"Call me T.J.," the celebrated surgeon said.

• ◆ •

Gernon grew up in the Pacific Northwest, an eighth-generation physician. He graduated from the University of Washington Medical School and later completed a prestigious five-year residency at the University of Michigan. But he never felt that his education and profession made him superior to the people he treated, or to anyone else. That value system had been instilled at a Jesuit high school that emphasized service to others. Gernon's mother was also a major influence.

"She is the embodiment of being a person for others," the surgeon said at City of Hope in 2019. "I always remember my mom saying you always evaluate somebody by how they treat the least person in the room. You never put yourself above anybody. Medicine is in my blood, but the trappings of being a doctor don't mean anything to me. I just do it because that's where I felt like I was guided to go. As far as asking patients to call me T.J., everyone is the same. I'm you, and you're me. I'm just a carpenter of the head and neck. Other guys are just as skilled at being plumbers. My job doesn't put me above anyone else."

Remarkably, he would find a version of that mindset in almost everyone he met in his new job. Humility was so common that it could have been a prerequisite to employment at City of Hope. It was not that way at many other major medical and research centers, where competition was fierce and where publication and recognition were often the measures of success. Many City of Hope clinicians and researchers had worked at places where ambition overshadowed a desire to serve.

"The well-being of patients seemed almost secondary the more powerful the individual was," said Dr. Joseph Alvarnas, a bone marrow and stem cell transplantation specialist, who came to City of Hope in 2008. He described places where he had trained and worked previously as "paradigms of deep human dysfunction and scientific greatness."

At City of Hope, Alvarnas found something altogether different: "When I came here, the thing that was most striking was that this was a community of people aligned in pursuit of something that was grounded, first and foremost, in honoring the humanity of the patients that we're privileged to serve. The second thing was the willingness to figuratively—and sometimes literally—hold the hands of patients for whom the best of medical care and the best of science was simply inadequate to the task they faced. And the third thing was a sense that this was a *community*, rather than a place where individual superstars would shine. And part of what was so striking is that the leaders walk the walk. They breathe the words and they lead by example."

But in 2016, City of Hope remained relatively unknown, even to Gernon. It had been "that place in Los Angeles." That modest public profile, Gernon said, "leads you to be, when you first come here, a little skeptical of other people and their training. But repeatedly, I found that the people I worked with trained at Stanford, or Michigan, or Harvard, MD Anderson, Sloan-Kettering—the best cancer centers in the country."

At City of Hope, Gernon discovered that the focus isn't on getting ahead, but on patients like Fred Claire. Like Fred, half of them arrive on the campus desperate because medical treatments had failed in other places.

"This is a place where patients come when they've had recurrences, when they've had defeats somewhere else, when they've had advanced disease and are looking for the penultimate treatment," said Dr. Ellie Maghami, a surgeon and director of the head and neck department at City of Hope. "They've already been so weathered and tested by everything else they've been through. By the time they get to us they are just really frail. They are very emotional. It's difficult. There is a lot that they need to process. There is a lot that we need to process and all this stuff is very delicate. Some of it is very similar from patient to patient. But some of it is very different from patient to patient. It's just a work environment that requires the kind of people who can provide that level of empathy and, I want to say, stubborn care. It means that you're tireless and you push forward and do whatever it takes. It takes that special physician to want to come to City of Hope. That kind of speaks to T.J."

A prominent example of City of Hope collegiality is the tumor board, where clinicians and researchers from a variety of specialties and disciplines convene to discuss the best course of treatment for an individual patient. Both Gernon and oncologist Dr. Erminia Massarelli were members of Fred Claire's board.

"Every single one of those people really embodies what we're talking about," Gernon said. "We're all on the same page with how we treat patients. Patients come first."

In tumor board meetings and in interactions with patients, there is also an unmistakable sense of urgency, one befitting a battle against a deadly foe. In cancer cases, Gernon said, "the doctor-patient relationship is different. Your backs are against the wall. You really have to fight for somebody. If you don't fight for somebody, they are not going to get better. If you're in this for the wrong reasons, if you're in this for the salary or the lifestyle, then you're not in it for the right reasons."

Fred Claire's back was certainly against the wall, and Gernon was blunt in his first meeting with his new patient. Fred Claire had a "nasty cancer," and his prognosis was grim. In cases of squamous cell carcinoma of the head, when the initial surgery does not eradicate the disease, less than one in four people are still alive five years later.

The surgeon described how a nerve that ran from Claire's lip to his jawbone and teeth, providing sensation to each of those areas, had become an expressway for the cancer that had originated in the lip.

"The tumor started to track back along the nerve into the jawbone, and he started having all this jaw pain," Gernon later recalled. "He was complaining to his dentist of all this pain in his teeth before he came to see me. When I saw him, I could feel a lump on the outside of the jawbone, which raised my suspicions. We did some imaging, and it showed that the nerve was really fat [with cancer] all the way to the jawbone."

Gernon offered Fred two choices. The most radical option, which the surgeon recommended, was called a sectional mandibulectomy, the removal of the cancerous section of jaw, which would be replaced with bone taken from the patient's leg. That offered the best chance of a cure, though certainly no guarantees. He and Fred had extensive discussions. The one worry Gernon had was that the tumor was still tracking on the nerve where he couldn't reach it. He didn't know if taking out the jawbone would necessarily make any difference in Fred's overall treatment.

In any event, Fred felt that such an invasive operation and the long healing it required might compromise the quality of whatever life he might have left. As an alternative, Gernon proposed a still difficult but somewhat less invasive procedure that involved drilling that nerve out of the jawbone, tracing it back as far as possible, cleaning the jawbone up and removing the lymph nodes. That was the surgeon's compromise.

Fred agreed, and the surgery was scheduled for October 14.

"T.J. made it very clear that this surgery wasn't going to be easy," Fred remembered. "In fact, he said you may or may not be able to feel your tongue afterward. This may be limiting. I don't know how long the surgery lasted, but when I came out, I said to Sheryl, 'I can move my tongue.'"

• ◆ •

For the next two months, City of Hope became a second home to the Claires while Fred underwent thirty-three radiation treatments and weekly chemotherapy. A woman named Lupe Santana was Fred's patient navigator, the person who met the Claires on one of their first visits to help them decipher the confusing labyrinth of the campus.

"Fred and Sheryl caught on quickly," Lupe said. "But on every visit I'd stop by and see them, wherever they were."

That is the City of Hope way.

Years before, while considering a job at the medical center, Lupe visited the Golter Gate and remembers her reaction. "I thought, 'If this place runs with that in mind, it will be a great place to work.' And it was true. Everybody here is willing to help you. Patients become navigators. If they see someone with that lost look, they'll say, 'Can I help you? Where are you going?' The culture is really what has kept me here."

Lupe had also personally witnessed one of the medical miracles that had become routine on the campus. Her sister, Olga

Rosas, had been diagnosed years before with breast cancer.

"Her doctor told her to go home and put her affairs in order," Lupe said. "He said, 'You have the most aggressive form of breast cancer there is, and no one survives this.'"

Olga then sought a second opinion from Dr. George Somlo at City of Hope.

"He said, 'I know what that is, and I know how to treat it,'" Lupe said. "He was researching inflammatory breast cancer, and he had a clinical trial available for her. It literally saved her life. If she had not come here for a second opinion, she would not be alive. She's going on her fourteenth year of being cancer-free."

Despite the anguish of Fred's serious diagnosis, he and his wife soon came to view City of Hope as a sanctuary, and people like Lupe Santana were among the main reasons why. Lupe, in fact, was the first person at the medical center with whom Fred shared his idea for a benefit golf tournament.

"I said to myself, 'I'm getting all the help. What is it that I can do?'" Fred recalled. "I said to Lupe, 'I've had this thought. I have enough contacts that we can have a golf tournament to raise money for City of Hope.'"

By late 2016, the medical news was also encouraging. Fred had surgery on October 14, finished chemo, and underwent his last radiation treatment on December 22. By January, he felt fighting fit. "I felt I had won the lottery," he said. But in the story of his journey at City of Hope, there would be many more difficult chapters to come.

4

HISTORY IN THE MAKING

The Dodgers lost their first four games of the 1987 season and seemed headed to another defeat in the fifth, trailing the San Francisco Giants by a run in the ninth inning. As the game began, the newly acquired Mickey Hatcher had been in the office of general manager Fred Claire, signing his contract. Hatcher had to rush to the clubhouse afterward to get into uniform.

Just minutes after making his way to the dugout, with the game on the line in the ninth, Dodgers manager Tommy Lasorda summoned Hatcher to pinch hit. His routine grounder went through the legs of the opposing third baseman, Chris Brown, allowing the tying run to score from third. As Dodger Stadium erupted, Claire got a call in his box.

"Are you having any fun?" Peter O'Malley asked him.

"Peter, we're going to win the pennant!" Claire shouted in reply.

However, the Hollywood ending would have to wait. The Giants went on to win the game in eleven innings, and the

Dodgers' season scarcely improved from there. For the second straight year, the team finished sixteen games under .500, a jarring reversal of fortune for the franchise that, between the years of 1952 and 1981, had won twelve National League pennants and five World Series championships.

"Oh, For Those Glory Days of Yesteryear," read a late-summer headline in *Sports Illustrated*. In the lengthy article that accompanied it, writer Peter Gammons noted that the Dodgers were destined to suffer consecutive losing seasons for the first time in nineteen years: "The realization was settling in that Dodger Blue is now the Dodger blues, a different state of mind entirely."

Gammons went on to describe a confounding ineptitude that included three errors in a single inning by the team's shortstop, Mariano Duncan, who then doffed his cap to the crowd and asked to be removed from the game, complaining of a migraine headache. Duncan was quickly demoted to the minors. One of the team's stars, Pedro Guerrero, insisted on coming out of the lineup because of intense booing by the home fans. In one game, three Dodger relief pitchers attempted to warm up at the same time, though there were only two available mounds in the bullpen. Gammons suggested that the entire organization was in similar disarray.

But rather than become discouraged, the embarrassing struggles and public broadsides only served to heighten Claire's resolve. Night after night during that season, Sheryl Claire woke in the wee hours to see her husband's side of the bed empty. She would find him in his home office, making notes or calls to baseball officials in other time zones.

"He wasn't going to back down once Peter [O'Malley] asked him to take the job," Sheryl Claire remembered. "Once he had it, he was never going to give it back unless it was taken from him. He didn't have enough time to do everything he wanted to do, but he loved every minute of it. That's just Fred."

But Claire also knew that his determination might not be enough to save his job. Soon after the season ended, he and O'Malley, the team owner and president, sat down for lunch at the Los Angeles Country Club.

"Peter told me he appreciated the dedication I had shown in replacing Al at the beginning of 1987, but he wanted me to know he was thinking of bringing in a 'more experienced' general manager," Claire recalls in *My 30 Years in Dodger Blue*. "I told Peter I could understand his thinking on this subject, but I had treasured every minute I had served as the GM and I wanted to continue in that capacity."

If O'Malley made a change, Claire also hinted he might not remain in the Dodger organization.

"I may go fly fishing in Montana for a while," Claire said, surprising his boss.

The club owner eventually did make serious inquiries about the availability of another general manager.

"Did I look at other possibilities? The answer is yes," O'Malley remembered in 2019. "However, the structure and the people we had in place in the baseball department, whether it was scouting or the minor leagues or player development, had been with us a long time, and it was a talented core of people. If you bring in somebody else, there is extraordinary turnover from top to bottom. I thought that the turmoil of complete change was a big negative. I didn't want to turn the organization upside down. I thought that would be a big mistake. And looking at Fred, whom I had known at the time for probably twenty years, it was not a difficult choice."

In early October of 1987, O'Malley announced that Claire and manager Tommy Lasorda would return in the same roles the following season. The next day, Claire rolled up his sleeves.

Working with a brain trust that included Lasorda and the Dodgers' major and minor league scouting departments, Claire began to evaluate his roster from top to bottom. Claire's collegiality and attention to detail became his trademarks, as he relied heavily on veteran professional scouts Mel Didier, Phil Regan, Steve Boros, and Jerry Stephenson.

"It was so easy to talk to Fred," Regan remembered in 2019. "When he talked to you, you got the feeling that he was interested in you, so it was really easy to give him reports. And he wanted to hear things. There was never anything too small about a player he was interested in. If we were going to make a trade, he would say, 'Does anyone know this player? Who do we know who has played with him? Who do we know who has coached him? How about his college coaches?' We went as far back as college to see what kind of a person this player was, how he would fit in on the team, his work habits. Fred wrote everything down and was organized. And he would value your opinion. He asked for it before he did anything."

Regan added, "Fred always said, 'They may have more talent, but they will never outwork us.' That was probably true. And he was much tougher than a lot of people perceived. He stood up to people. When he believed in something, he didn't back down. He would listen to you, but he made up his own mind."

The discussion among Claire and his advisors centered on several areas of obvious need. One priority was finding a shortstop who could catch the ball and solidify the infield; another was bringing in a reliable closer to finish off games. Claire and his brain trust pored over statistics and scouting reports, looking for players on other teams who might help patch up the team's most glaring deficiencies. Claire also evaluated potential players in less tangible ways.

"Right off the bat, Fred got in touch with what the Dodgers were always about: that is character people and character players," said Mike Scioscia, a Dodger catcher at the time who went on to become the long-time manager of the Los Angeles Angels. "He put a lot of weight on what players were like in the clubhouse, off the field, how hard they played."

Mickey Hatcher, who had been released by the Minnesota Twins in the spring of 1987, was one example. Another was outfielder John Shelby, who Claire snatched out of Baltimore's minor league system. Veteran catcher Rick Dempsey was a third.

By the time he showed up outside Fred Claire's office in the winter of 1987, Dempsey was thirty-eight years old and had played eighteen years in the major leagues. But he was not ready to retire. Dempsey waited for hours outside Claire's office until the general manager emerged in the early evening.

"Fred, I've never quit at anything in my life," Dempsey said. "Just give me a couple of minutes of your time. If it doesn't work out, no worries, no hard feelings. I can retire if I want."

Claire invited him in and listened.

"This is what I'll do," Dempsey said. "I'll hit a home run every twenty-five at bats. We will take this pitching staff, and we'll turn it around. We'll win our division, win the playoffs. We'll get into the World Series. We'll win the World Series. I'll catch the last pitch, and I'll give you the ball."

Claire was impressed by the passion that still burned in the veteran player, particularly after the dismal and painful season in Cleveland that Dempsey had just endured. His batting average had been .177, and his season was ended by a jarring home plate collision with the massive former football star, Bo Jackson.

"You're invited to spring training," Claire told Dempsey as the meeting concluded.

It would turn out to be one of the most memorable seasons of Dempsey's long career. Decades later, Dempsey said that the Dodger general manager was a major reason why: "When I met Fred, I thought, here's a guy who believed just like I did, that we could win no matter what. When Fred talked about this ball club and the belief he had in these players, I think he made us all believe, and that's a gift. There are not many people in the game of baseball that could do that. You've got to give Tommy Lasorda credit, but Fred was the one really that put that team together and when he talked about the players that we had, there was so much conviction in his voice that these guys could win."

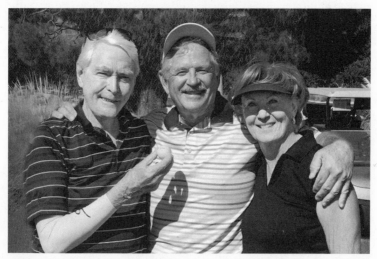

Thirty-two years after Rick Dempsey gave Fred the final out baseball of the 1988 World Series, Fred and Sheryl enjoyed a day of golf with Rick at Oakmont Country Club.

•◆•

The Winter Meetings of Major League Baseball general managers are part rumor mill and part flea market, times for bartering, negotiating and trade making. In the 1987 meetings, Claire made it known that he was ready to deal. But his colleagues quickly noticed that the new Dodger general manager went about his job much differently than his predecessor.

"I wouldn't say that arrogance preceded Fred, but I would say the Dodgers felt that they held a special place in the baseball firmament and that related to all things baseball," Sandy Alderson, the general manager of the Oakland A's at the time, said in a 2019 interview. "Working with Fred, obviously his experience in the game up to that point had not been specifically related to the game itself, development or scouting. But he had certainly absorbed a tremendous amount about the game, was very knowledgeable and capable.

"Fred also came armed with an engaging personality. Believe me, that goes a long way," Alderson said. "I think people genuinely liked him. People within the Dodger organization and people who had dealt with him in the LA media felt he was basically a nice guy, pleasant and respectful. Because of all those things, people gave him the benefit of the doubt, which everybody needs at the outset."

Alderson was Claire's partner in his first blockbuster trade. The Dodgers agreed to send Bob Welch, a young and much coveted starting pitcher, to the A's in exchange for shortstop Alfredo Griffin and reliever Jay Howell. This was part of a three-team trade that also involved the New York Mets and brought left-handed relief pitcher Jesse Orosco to the Dodgers.

The new players instantly plugged three of the Dodgers' most glaring holes.

Claire and the Dodgers then turned their attention to Detroit Tigers outfielder Kirk Gibson, a free agent that year. Gibson had also been an All-American football player at Michigan State, and he brought a gritty, gridiron mentality to baseball. In nine years with the Tigers, he had put up elite statistics for home runs, runs batted in, and stolen bases, but it was his attitude that Claire most coveted.

Claire had done his homework. He learned that a highly respected scout in Wisconsin, Dale McReynolds, had submitted stellar reports on Gibson going back to the player's college days.

"Dale was never one to go overboard on a player, but when I saw his reports on Kirk, I called him," Claire recalled years later. "Dale confirmed every glowing word he had put on paper."

Gibson's courtship would be the beginning of a relationship with Claire that endured for more than three decades but was not without its rocky moments.

"I had some great encounters with Fred over the years, but I always respected him, and he always respected me," Gibson remembered in 2019. "We actually grew closer through our disagreements. I remember one day with Fred and Tommy it got a little confrontational. Fred kind of raised his voice and said, 'Young man, you're not talking to Fred Claire. You're talking to the Dodgers.' I came right back and said, 'I don't care who I'm talking to.' He put his glasses on the top of his head and got in my face, and I got in his face. But you know what? I always loved Fred, his passion, and his delivery, and he never held it against me, either. I thought, 'This is the guy I want in my foxhole.'"

In the winter of 1988, O'Malley and Lasorda joined Claire in an all-out effort to lure Gibson to Southern California.

"They were very aggressive," Gibson recalled. "I was a Michigan boy, a Midwest boy, and so now you meet Fred, and what he represents, and you meet Tommy and you meet Peter O'Malley, and you go to Dodger Stadium and it's like, holy shit, it's Hollywood, you know? It's beautiful. It wasn't hard to sell that place. And very honestly, Fred, Tommy, and Peter O'Malley were very convincing."

Claire signed Gibson to a three-year contract. The two of them sat down to dinner shortly thereafter.

"I told Fred, 'I'm pretty serious, and I'm going to be intense. Don't be surprised. I might have to kick some ass,'" Gibson recalled. "I had won one World Series, and I wanted to win another. I didn't want to live in California to go to Hollywood. Fred said something like, 'Why do you think you're here?'"

• ◆ •

In his first nine big league seasons with the Tigers, Gibson had played for Hall of Fame manager Sparky Anderson.

"Sparky is . . . instead of saying strict, I'll say *structured*," Gibson said. "He would have these meetings in the spring before you go out on the field to go over what you're going to do. Maybe there was a joke or two, but nothing too big. Sparky was all business. He laid it out. 'We're going to do bunt plays today. Not only are you going to do them, but you're going to do them right.' His philosophy was, if you don't do them right in practice, what are you going to do in the ninth inning of a game?"

When Gibson reported to his first spring training with the Dodgers, he found a different atmosphere altogether: "Everyone was screwing around and it was real loud and they were all yelling at Tommy."

One day, clowns literally jumped out of equipment trunks that had been placed in the middle of the locker room. The jollity carried over onto the field. During a fielding drill, Dodgers star Pedro Guerrero picked up a ball and hurled it into the outfield.

"Everybody started laughing, and I thought, 'What's funny about that?'" Gibson recalled. "Quite frankly, I was a little nervous about our lack of focus. That went on every day."

Gibson, on the other hand, planned to play every preseason game like it was the seventh game of the World Series. The Dodgers' spring training opener was against the Japanese national team. During warmups, Gibson ran outfield sprints with an intensity that caused his hat to fly off. Teammates and spectators immediately began to laugh.

"Kirk couldn't understand the reaction until he reached up to his forehead and eye-black, that thick, greasy material used by athletes to deflect potentially blinding rays of the sun, came off in his hand," Claire wrote in his memoir.

A teammate had secretly spread the goo inside Gibson's cap, and now it was smeared across his face. Gibson snapped and left the field, making for the clubhouse. Lasorda asked Gibson to return, but he refused.

Newly acquired relief pitcher Jay Howell was in the Dodger clubhouse when Gibson came storming in and remembered him throwing his stuff in his locker and stripping off his uniform. "I thought, 'This ain't right,'" Howell recalled more than thirty years later. "I could see the eye-black and Gibson raising holy hell and yelling, 'No wonder you guys finished last.' I mean it went on and on and I was like, 'Whoa, what do we have here?'"

The memory also remained vivid for Gibson: "I told Tommy, 'Go get the bastard who did the eye-black.' I said, 'We've got clowns jumping out of the trunks. We do drills, and we're throwing it into right field and everybody is laughing. There is nothing funny about that.' That was just me being me. I'm taking no prisoners. I'm full go. Nobody knew that and nobody realized that. Tommy said, 'They're trying to make you feel welcome.' I said, 'I don't want to feel welcome. I want to win. I'm not looking for friends; I'm looking for people who get after it.' They wouldn't go get the guy, so I left."

Gibson met Lasorda and Claire early the next morning. The manager pleaded with his new star player to calm down, asking that when reporters questioned him, Gibson should attribute his absence the previous day to an unexpected family matter. The player refused: "I said, 'This is what's going to happen. Before the meeting, whoever did it needs to come up, and I'll talk to them. And secondly, when we have our meeting, I'll speak. Either this happens, or I'm out of here. Maybe I came to the wrong place.' I didn't care what happened. All I knew was that I was going to say what I had to say, and if they didn't like me, they could get rid of me. Either I had made a terrible mistake, or they were willing to change."

Relief pitcher Jesse Orosco confessed to the prank.

"I told Orosco, 'You know what, I'm the best teammate you've ever had, but you screw with me one more time, you won't pitch another inning in your life. Sorry man.'"

Then Gibson addressed the team: "I just stood up and I said, 'You guys are a bunch of losers. You've lost the last how many years? It's not hard to see why. You come in here and it's a big comedy show. Winning is what's fun to me.'"

Gibson saw jaws dropping as he looked around the room at his teammates.

"I can tell by the look on your faces that you don't know quite how to take me," he said. "But I will sacrifice for all of you in here."

Then he challenged his new teammates to a fight, all of them at once if need be.

"I'm not worried about that," he said. "What I'm worried about is you guys understanding how I am as your teammate. I may not be the toughest guy, but I'm crazy enough to believe I'm the toughest guy. We are going to be tough. We are going to get after their asses. Anybody who wants to get it on, let's go."

There were no takers.

"That was magnificent," Jay Howell recalled. "That was just theater. It was grand theater. I mean, I had visions of Clint Eastwood."

Claire later wrote, "After one game in the spring, Kirk Gibson had assumed control of the Dodger clubhouse."

"I don't think he took it over," O'Malley said. "I think the players gave it to him. I think the players had so much respect for him and what he stood for and what he was all about that he emerged naturally as the leader and led the team, with Orel Hershiser and others."

His teammates learned immediately that Gibson was not just talk.

"Every single day for the next six months he backed it up," said Tim Belcher, a rookie starting pitcher on the 1988 team.

More than three decades later, Belcher remembered that year's Opening Day. Early in the game, the Dodgers' second baseman, Steve Sax, led off an inning with a double.

"Before the ball was even thrown back into the infield, Gibson is on the top step of the dugout getting ready to go to the on-deck circle. And he's screaming at whoever it was that was hitting after Sax, screaming at the top of his lungs, 'Do your job! Get him over [to third]!' It scared the hell out of everybody, including Lasorda, who was standing right beside him. We're all looking at each other like, 'Oh my God.' It's the first game of the year in April, and this guy is already so intense. He did that all year. He backed it up."

Gibson would bat third in a lineup that included solid returnees like catcher Mike Scioscia, second baseman Steve Sax, and outfielder Mike Marshall, but no one would have confused the 1988 Dodgers batting order with the Murderer's Row of the 1927 New York Yankees. Yet there was a magic about the Dodgers that began to manifest itself in spring training. Game after game, players like Hatcher, Dave Anderson, and Dempsey, the self-proclaimed "Stuntmen," came off the bench in late innings of exhibitions to rally the team to victory.

"I had played on some fabulous teams in the course of my career, six divisional titles and three World Series, but that was by far the most fun anybody could have on a baseball team," Dempsey remembered.

Gibson said the team bonded in ways that exceeded even his expectations: "We were a team of pieces that collaborated, cooperated and were teammates to some special nth power. Fred built a team of players with a lot of character, who loved to play the game, and were good teammates. We were so complementary. We were his baby. Tommy [Lasorda] was masterful as well. Everything kept falling into place. People would say we weren't this or that and it didn't matter to us."

The Dodgers lost their season opener but then won five straight and never looked back, taking over first place for good in late May.

"After every game we won, I think it was Tommy who started it, he would come into the clubhouse and yell, 'What a bleeping team! How sweet it is!' By mid-year, after wins, we'd come in and everybody would be standing there, and I'd go, 'What a bleeping team. Oh yeah. How sweet it is! The fruits of victory!' And all the guys would join in."

Gibson would eventually be named the National League's Most Valuable Player. Star pitcher Orel Hershiser, who anchored a dominant starting rotation, set a league record for consecutive scoreless innings and won the National League Cy Young Award after one of the greatest seasons for a pitcher in baseball history. Jay Howell became the reliable closer that the team had lacked. Alfredo Griffin was masterful at shortstop, and John Shelby a defensive wizard in center. The late-inning magic of Hatcher, Dempsey, and the other Stuntmen came to epitomize the season.

"Through all of August and September, as we got closer to winning the division, the main thought I had was how great this was going to be for the Dodger organization," Claire remembered in 2019. "We had been through such a tough period. I thought, 'If we continue on here, I'm going to have a chance to speak on behalf of the organization, saying the Dodgers are back where they belong as a contending team. And I'm going to acknowledge so many who rarely receive acknowledgment: our scouts, player development personnel, our medical team, and the major league staff."

The Dodgers clinched a tie for the division championship against the Giants in late September. In the celebration afterward, someone handed Claire a squirt gun, which he used to douse nearby players and coaches—highly uncharacteristic frivolity for the general manager.

A few days later, against the Padres in San Diego, Mickey Hatcher's eighth-inning single drove in the winning run, ensuring a division title for the team that had been a laughingstock the year before.

"They really believed," a jubilant Lasorda said after the game. "I really believed."

The Dodgers finished the season with ninety-four victories, twenty-one more than each of the two previous years. Fred Claire was later named Major League Baseball's Executive of the Year, joining Dodger legends who had won the same award previously, like Larry MacPhail, Branch Rickey, Walter O'Malley, and Buzzie Bavasi.

"It was such an effort of everybody coming together," Claire said. "There was tremendous satisfaction and joy and excitement and momentum. Here's a team with a mixture of guys like Scioscia and Steve Sax and Mike Marshall and Orel, who had been through two terrible seasons. But we were going back to the playoffs. There was a realization that we had something here."

Most outside the Dodgers' clubhouse inner circle believed the feel-good story was destined for an unhappy ending. They would face the New York Mets in the National League playoffs. The two teams had played eleven times during the regular season; the Mets had won ten.

"They had kicked our butts pretty good," Fred Claire conceded years later. "But there was clearly no intimidation, no fear. I certainly didn't think, 'Oh, we've come this far, but now we're overmatched.' There was never that sense."

5

A DIFFERENT BALLGAME
NOW

By late February 2017, Fred and Sheryl Claire believed that the agonies of cancer were behind them. Though exhausted over the holidays—his body depleted by surgery, chemotherapy, and radiation—Fred's energy gradually returned in January. By the following month, he and his wife had returned to a normal life.

Fred was once again strong enough to shoulder his golf bag. He had resumed his weekly breakfasts with friends at the venerable Pasadena eatery called Pie 'n Burger. On Tuesday, February 21, 2017, after what was to be a routine checkup with Dr. Gernon, the couple planned to drive to their vacation home in the California desert.

"We felt we were sailing in clear skies," Fred Claire recalled.

Anxiety accompanies any cancer checkup, but given Fred's increasingly robust health, Sheryl expected Gernon to merely confirm what they already believed.

"We just thought we were going in to have everybody say, 'Everything is great. You look good,'" Sheryl Claire remembered. "In fact, when we walked in, T.J. said, 'You look great.' We felt great. We thought that we were in the clear, but that day changed everything."

After a brief chat with the couple, Gernon began to prod Fred's neck with his fingers. The physician's demeanor abruptly changed.

"I don't like this," he said. "Don't you feel this?"

"T.J., my neck is so stiff and sore from radiation, I don't feel anything at all," Fred replied.

Gernon had discovered a lump and knew immediately that it could mean only one thing. The cancer had returned. The doctor's stomach sank, and he told the Claires, "We're going to have to do something, *now*."

For several moments, the Claires sat in devastated silence.

"Early on, we just never could get a break, never got anything positive. Never got anything good," Sheryl remembered. "Then when this came back, it was like—that's the problem: You think you feel good, you think you're getting back to normal and you're going to have your life back, and then cancer just pulls the rug right out from under you. It was kind of like it was going, 'Ha. Ha. Ha. I'm back.'"

Fred said, "In the beginning, T.J. had called it a nasty cancer with a 20 percent survival rate, and now the diagnosis had gotten worse. Not only was it in my jaw. Now it was in my neck. Here you are, physically you feel in good shape and mentally you are in good shape, but something is taking control of your body. That something is cancer."

Gernon immediately scheduled a series of tests. Fred was at

home a few days later when the call came.

"That was the darkest day of all," he remembered. "We were in a room upstairs when we got the call. It was T.J. saying that the squamous cell carcinoma that I had in my jaw was now in my neck. I knew that this was a different ballgame now. It just didn't look good. Then in the follow-up meetings, they told us they couldn't do any more radiation. They couldn't do any more chemotherapy. They couldn't operate again."

•◆•

On February 17, 2017, four days before the world of Fred and Sheryl Claire abruptly took a dire turn, a close friend named Rich Kee left a package on the front porch of their Pasadena home. He called Fred and told him to look for the delivery.

"What is it?" Fred asked.

"I can't tell you now," Kee said. "You'll understand later. But don't open the box until Sheryl is home. Open it later in the evening when you are done with your day and have time to enjoy what's in it."

Fred agreed to wait.

"He probably thought it was a bottle of wine," Kee laughed later.

Forty-one years before, Kee had been a young photographer with a love of baseball and a dream. He wrote to Fred, then a marketing executive with the Dodgers, asking for an audition to be the team photographer. Fred agreed to let Kee shoot a handful of games at Dodger Stadium.

"I came up with a multimedia slide presentation with photos and music, based on the games that Fred allowed me to photograph," Kee remembered. "I set that up in the boardroom at

Dodger Stadium and went back to Fred's office and told him it was ready. He said, 'Let's do it right now.'"

Kee was excited, and his heart started to thunder.

"You have to remember, I'm a young kid in awe of Dodger Stadium and nervous as hell. We were walking down the hallway to the boardroom and Fred stopped. He said, 'Hold on for a minute, Rich.' He leaned into the open door of Peter O'Malley's office and said, 'Peter, I want you to see something.' I will never forget that compliment of including Peter in the presentation without even seeing an image."

The team owner joined them in the boardroom.

"He and Fred sat there and saw the presentation," Kee said. "To this day, it's one of my greatest memories. Peter said, 'Can I see it one more time?' That was the beginning of my stay at Dodger Stadium."

Fred and Rich became close friends during the photographer's eight years with the team and remained so in the decades that followed. In the fall and early winter of 2016, like so many of Fred's friends, Kee wrestled with a sense of helplessness after learning of the catastrophic cancer diagnosis: "You're sitting there watching this play out in front of you. I wracked my brain, wondering what I could do to bring some reassurance or something positive to him. Then the idea came to me."

Kee composed an email, which he sent to scores of people, informing them of Fred's battle with jaw cancer and asking for contributions to be part of a special gift: a large hardcover book containing a collection of shared experiences or words of encouragement from colleagues Fred had enjoyed during his Dodger years and beyond. Kee asked for contributions that were "positive, memorable, and smile makers." Since the project was time sensitive, Kee set a seven-day deadline. Most responses came within two.

From Pete Rose:

I just did a little arithmetic and figured out I must have played in 1,781 away games, a [MLB] record as an active player. Hundreds of those games were at Dodger Stadium, a baseball shrine where Fred Claire's contributions to the Dodger traditions of class and winning are up there on the same pedestal as Koufax, Garvey, and Lasorda.

From Steve Garvey:

There are those who have style and those who have class. But, once in a while, those two great virtues are embedded in a single person. Fred Claire is that kind of man. And I am honored to call him my friend.

Longtime baseball executive Peter Bavasi wrote:

One of your many attributes, Fred, is that with all your many successes over the years, you have not changed at all. You remain the most decent, thoughtful and caring of baseball people. [. . .] You have touched the lives of thousands of ballplayers, and young front-office aspirants, and umpires; and writers and broadcasters, too. You shared with us your optimism and enthusiasm and belief that we could achieve anything we put our hard work into. You always had a kind word of encouragement for those who needed it most. [. . .] You set an example for treating everyone with thoughtfulness, decency, loyalty, and care.

From Dodger pitching legend Orel Hershiser:

Any time a player needed a little more help, Fred made sure they got what they needed. Personal advice was not beyond his reach either, and it extended from helping me evaluate my home purchase in Pasadena to touring houses and helping with appraisals. [. . .] He is passionate, caring, competitive, and one of the best role models anyone could have. A Dodger in the truest sense, like Jackie [Robinson], Sandy [Koufax], and others, he is one of the best!!

But the vast majority of the seventy-six responses came from people unrecognizable to the general public.

"I wanted the book to be not only a mixture of high-profile folks but also everyday people who were off the public radar," Kee said later. "Fred doesn't measure his friends by public popularity. Everybody is equal. I thought the book needed to be a combination of people in his life, high and low profile."

One of Kee's favorite examples was Merri Ann Irons, a longtime waitress at Pie 'n Burger. For many years, Fred and his friends had insisted on sitting at the table where Irons would take their orders and serve their food. She was dumbstruck when Kee asked her to contribute to the book.

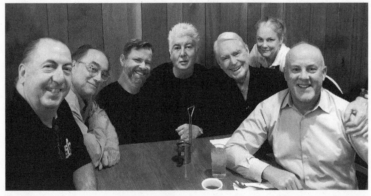

Fred's breakfast hangout has been Pie 'n Burger in Pasadena. Here, he visits with longtime friends (from left) Paige Parrish, Michael Trim, Mark Goodstein, Rich Kee, and Todd Derrick, as waitress and friend Merri Ann Irons looks on.

"She said to me, 'Are you telling me I'm going to be in a book with Orel Hershiser?'" Kee said. "I said, 'Absolutely, Merri Ann. Why would you ask me that? Don't you think you're entitled to be in there? Fred thinks as much of you as he does Orel.'"

Irons wrote that she always called Fred the "wild card" because, after all the years of serving him, she could never predict what he would order. Her tribute read:

> In twenty years of serving customers, I can't think of a finer gentleman and friend. Your humility and kindness to me and the rest of the staff here is one of the many reasons why we're so happy to see you walk through that door. [. . .] Fred, above all, what I admire most is your absolute love and dedication to Sheryl. You both are very special individuals to me, and I am so proud that you two would consider me your friend. Hurry, get well. [. . .] I miss you.

Kee added his own tribute before having a single copy of the book printed for the Claires. It read:

> When this once-skinny kid first stepped onto the manicured grass of Dodger Stadium forty-one years ago, with a Nikon stuck to his forehead, I had no idea what I was in store for. Little did I know that down the road, the one I would admire and be most influenced by was not a player in uniform, but a gentleman upstairs with an office overlooking one very storied front lawn. Fred, because of you and your confidence in me, I have amassed a lifetime of cherished memories.

Rich Kee's unopened package was on the kitchen table when Sheryl returned home that night. Fred had been waiting. The couple opened the box to find an exquisite coffee-table book with a close-up photograph of a baseball on the white cover, the red stitching in tight focus.

Below the ball's seam was the one-word title, "Shared." The first page contained Kee's short introduction:

What you will find in the pages ahead are friends and colleagues from 913 E. California [the address of Pie 'n Burger] to 25 Main [the address of the Baseball Hall of Fame in Cooperstown, New York] and all over and in-between. Folks have reached out to express their heartfelt best wishes and, at the same time, share with you the impact you've had on their lives along the way. It's a small sampling from your vast library of friends, ones that wanted to remind you they care. Enjoy, Mr. Claire . . . enjoy.

Fred and Sheryl turned the page to see the first message from Paige Parrish, Fred's friend and longtime lawyer. Hershiser's was next. A celebrity wrote on one page, a clubhouse attendant at the Claires' country club on another. The couple was stunned by the succession of names and the litany of heartfelt comments. Fred thought it may have been the best gift he had ever received.

"We were just amazed," Sheryl said later. "We had obviously no idea Rich had done this. We felt such gratitude that people would respond and had such wonderful things to say about Fred, and for the outpouring of love."

Fred called Kee.

"Rich, this is going to be a short call, because we've just started to read the book," Fred said, his voice thick with emotion. "That's all I can say."

Every page brought a cherished memory.

"A wonderful thing about Rich's book is the variety of people, of friendships, of relationships," Fred remembered later. "For someone to take the time to do that was just so meaningful. Reading messages from young people who started with the Dodgers, people I hadn't heard from in fifteen or twenty years, carried as much meaning as someone with celebrity status. It was quite overwhelming. The support of others is truly a powerful healing tool. It was an unforgettable gift."

• ◆ •

Just four days later, in an examination room at City of Hope, came the terrible news. Fred and Sheryl tried to soldier on.

"I don't remember thinking the end was near, that he would not survive this," Sheryl recalled. "That was unthinkable. I think we geared up for the next battle."

But something profound had shifted for them both.

"It was a mental game changer," Fred remembered. "When you have that type of news as a patient, you have to adjust to the reality that, very frankly, the end could be near. You have to be realistic and accept what you're being told. After that, Sheryl and I would take many walks, and there was clearly a different tone to what we were talking about: 'Let's enjoy this walk. Let's just enjoy this walk.' It wasn't, 'When are we going to the desert?' or making plans to go here or there. It was two people and their families coming together and saying, 'We could be facing something that is not life changing, but life ending.'"

One night at home, the cruel realities caught up with Sheryl. She had gone into a bedroom to change clothes after the couple had been out to dinner. "I can remember just collapsing on the bed, just sobbing uncontrollably," she said. "I was just realizing what we're dealing with, knowing what life had been like together, and the thought that it may not continue. Was it fear? I honestly don't know. I just know it was this uncontrollable sobbing."

Fred was determined to push on in his trademark manner.

"Cancer treatments are like a baseball season—you don't win the pennant or lose it in one single day," he said. "You keep giving your best every day, with focus and discipline, and try not to react to anything on an emotional basis. It's a matter of believing in the people around you who are doing their best to assist. Sorry to get carried away with a baseball analogy, but the game provides lessons on getting through a long season and staying focused while always giving your best."

But for the first time, Fred had been forced to come to terms with the fact that his ultimate season might be coming to an end.

"It's not that I went into depression and gave up," he continued. "But if you get a diagnosis like that, I think mentally we were preparing for the reality of life and the reality of death. Mortality."

And just a few years earlier, the recurrence of his cancer would have been just that—a death sentence.

6

MAKINGS OF A MIRACLE

I t was impossible to pinpoint the spark of the cosmic chain reaction, the confluence of vision and resources, perseverance and serendipity, that ultimately led to Fred Claire's medical miracle.

There were many possible beginnings. One came in the 1990s, in the California laboratory of a young researcher named James Allison. He was a shaggy-haired, harmonica-playing, free spirit from Texas who made the study of T cells—the human body's disease- and infection-fighting white blood cells—his life's work. With the loss of several relatives to cancer, including his mother and brother, Allison turned his focus to fighting the disease.

He and other researchers sought the answer to one of the most puzzling and stubborn riddles of medical science: Why were T cells, which so efficiently attacked infection and many types of diseases, so ineffectual when it came to cancer?

Saul Priceman, a researcher who came to City of Hope in 2010, said, "When I was doing my Ph.D. studies, I was one of the very few people at UCLA, and maybe in the nation, who was saying, 'We should be co-opting the immune system [in the fight against cancer].' Very few people were saying that if you could teach the immune system to see cancer, it should do it well and continue to do it in a very durable way. It does so against viruses and other pathogens, why not against cancer? But for whatever reason, the immune system that houses your best army in fighting cancer is defective in cancer patients."

In his lab at the University of California at Berkeley, Allison, simultaneously with another scientist, made a discovery that suggested an answer: isolating a protein molecule on the surface of the T cell. The molecule's purpose was to rein in the T cell. Called a checkpoint, it would shut down the cell if it became over exuberant and began to attack healthy cells and tissue in addition to viruses and pathogens.

But researchers discovered that checkpoint molecules were also a major ally of cancer. Through a complicated biological process, cancer cells tricked the checkpoints into incapacitating T cells, thereby suppressing the immune system when it was needed most. Cancer was thus free to proliferate without the resistance of the body's primary disease-fighting mechanism. Clearly, in cases of cancer, the checkpoints themselves needed to be neutralized. But how?

Allison and a graduate student came up with the answer by developing an antibody that would disarm the checkpoint. Thus unshackled, the soldiers of the immune system could join the fight against cancer.

A 2016 story in the *New York Times* reported: "When researchers gave the antibody to mice with cancer, tumors vanished. Recalling those first tests in mice, Dr. Allison said it was astounding to see the cancers shrink and disappear. Veterinarians thought the mice had contracted an infection or a skin disease. But the sores that worried the vets were actually tumors that were ulcerating and rotting away under assault by T cells."

The *Times* story added: "Many drug companies were skeptical about the findings, but one, Medarex, created a human version of the antibody. The antibody, given the trade name Yervoy, was approved in 2011 to treat advanced melanoma. It became the first drug to prolong survival of people with this deadly form of cancer."

Other early results in humans were similarly astounding. After receiving what became known as checkpoint inhibitors, studies showed that one-in-five patients in the final stages of cancer were alive three years later, many apparently cancer-free.

It was the beginning of a revolution in cancer treatment, which heretofore had relied almost exclusively on surgery, chemotherapy, and radiation. Following Allison's breakthrough, scores of different checkpoint inhibitors were developed and tested in hundreds of clinical trials. Many were proven to be remarkably effective in combating solid tumors in the body.

Researchers around the world were simultaneously exploring another means of unleashing the body's immune system against cancer. In what became known as CAR [chimeric antigen receptor] T cell therapy, a patient's T cells were extracted from the blood and supercharged in a laboratory. An antigen called a CAR was added to the T cells, which programmed them to identify and attack cancer. CAR T cell therapy was proven to be particularly effective in treating blood cancers like leukemia, and lymphoma.

Immunotherapy worked for only one-in-five patients, and researchers around the world raced to understand why. But by 2016, when Fred Claire's battle with the disease began, the combination of checkpoint inhibitors and CAR T had made the miraculous increasingly commonplace. Thousands of patients who would have died just a few years before enjoyed long and often cancer-free reprieves. One prominent example is President Jimmy Carter, who was diagnosed in 2015 with melanoma that had spread to his brain, a condition that just a few years before would have almost certainly been fatal. A year later, after immunotherapy was brought to bear against his disease, Carter announced he no longer needed treatment.

Dr. Steven Rosen, a City of Hope oncologist and researcher who specializes in blood diseases, said, "In my domain, there is not a single patient that I see where in my mind, I don't think we can't control the disease. We're not always successful, but it's been such a dramatic change. In the last year and a half, I have not had a single death. Going back, I was regularly attending funerals for my patients."

In 2018, James Allison was one of two immunotherapy researchers awarded the Nobel Prize for medicine. By then he headed the immunology department at the famed MD Anderson Cancer Center in Houston. One of his protégés there was a young oncologist and researcher from Italy, Dr. Erminia Massarelli. She would eventually lead the fight for Fred Claire's life.

•◆•

Robert Stone grew up in Southern California, but until the 1990s had only a passing familiarity with City of Hope. In 1996, as a young graduate of the University of Chicago Law School, he resisted attempts by the medical center to recruit him for its legal team.

"Then I received a phone call that changed my life. I grew up and spent my early years within fifteen miles of City of Hope's campus. I knew the organization did great work, but I hadn't been touched by cancer at that point in my life. And so, when City of Hope called me in 1996 to see if I might be interested in working there, I said no. In fact, I told them no twice.

"But I agreed to an interview, and I then took a tour of the campus. We were walking past the pediatric bone marrow transplant unit. Just outside the building, I spotted a nurse pulling a little red wagon. Inside the red wagon was a bald-headed child. The child was smiling, beaming intense enjoyment just to be outside in the sunlight. But I'll tell you what really grabbed my heart: Right behind the wagon was the child's mother, pushing a pole with the IV bag and silently sobbing. And it was clear to me that these were not tears of sorrow, but tears of joy as she saw her child enjoying the sunshine—and knowing there would be many more days of sunshine ahead.

"It was at that instant I decided to say yes.

"That was one of the luckiest days of my life. I wanted to be part of this special place that developed highly advanced treatments . . . put those treatments into practice . . . and took patients for rides in little red wagons."

Over the next two decades, Stone would hold eleven different positions at City of Hope, culminating with his appointment as president in 2012 and CEO two years later. He inherited the legacy of Samuel Golter and Ben Horowitz. Like his predecessors, Stone became a compelling evangelist for the humanitarian values upon which City of Hope was founded.

But his vision for the institution went far beyond the perpetuation of its trademark humility and compassion. Stone seemed determined to prove that a medical center could be both a model for humanity and the tip of the scientific spear when it came to the fight against disease.

In 2012, Ashley Baker Lee joined City of Hope to lead research operations. Years later, she recalled an early conversation with Stone:

"He said, 'Ashley, in five years, this is where I want to be,'" Stone told her. "I want to be a top-five comprehensive cancer center.' He really was the one that set those targets. He believed in that vision and was the one that articulated them."

But Stone needed someone to translate that vision into reality, and by 2014 the search for the right person seemed to have stalled. That was when City of Hope executives got wind of Dr. Steven Rosen's transition after twenty-five years as the leader of the prestigious cancer center at Northwestern University. Rosen had grown weary of the constant pressures of grant seeking at the behemoth educational institution.

"It was serendipitous," Rosen recalled. "I had announced that I was going to step down from my position at Northwestern, thinking I'd still stay there and do something else. They [City of Hope executives] heard about it and contacted me."

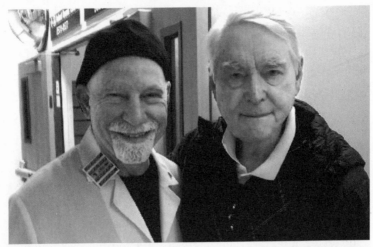

Dr. Steven Rosen is the provost and chief scientific officer at City of Hope. In addition to directing the Comprehensive Cancer Center, Rosen leads the Beckman Research Institute at City of Hope.

Rosen initially could not envision living on the West Coast, but the fact that three of Rosen's four children were living in California, as were his parents, inspired him to at least consider it. "Until then, I didn't appreciate the physical beauty of this area, nor did I appreciate the foundation that existed at City of Hope that could be built upon," Rosen said. "When I came out, I saw the physical beauty, the unique campus, and the infrastructure. This was a hundred-year-old operation, but in some ways, it was still in its infancy."

He felt there was much that was special about City of Hope, the place where Stephen Forman, one of Rosen's heroes, had practiced for decades. "But it really was Steve and a few other people," Rosen said. But at City of Hope, there were financial resources to change that, in part due to the royalties from Arthur Riggs' discoveries. Rosen decided to move west to become City of Hope's provost and chief scientific officer, and he aggressively embraced Stone's vision.

Ashley Baker Lee said, "Dr. Rosen said to Robert Stone, 'I need to recruit fifty top people. Here are the areas that I need to build strength in.' He went for the best in the country. Robert spent hundreds of millions in recruitment."

That investment meant that the American medical world, witnessing the procession of talent to Duarte, soon began to buzz.

"I was a cancer center director at Northwestern for twenty-five years," Rosen said. "I was familiar with what you need to do, and I knew everyone in the field. People trust me. They like me. We put together competitive packages for top people and then attracted people who were extraordinarily talented coming out of their training. I started recruiting some stars. You recruit two or three stars, and the next thing you know, everyone wants to come."

Rosen pursued clinicians and researchers he knew and admired, but also those who would fit the City of Hope culture.

"We are always looking for an individual who has the intellectual talent, the work ethic, but also is empathetic and wears on their sleeve the desire to essentially follow what Samuel Golter said decades ago about humanitarianism, service and reward," Rosen said. "That's the kind of person we recruit. Every person I recruit is someone I'd like to have a beer or a glass of wine with."

Rosen soon persuaded Dr. Yuman Fong, one of the world's leading cancer surgeons and researchers, to leave the renowned Memorial Sloane-Kettering Cancer Center in New York City, where Fong had worked for two decades. He became the head of surgery at City of Hope.

"He's maybe the most gifted clinician/scientist I've ever met," Rosen said. "As a robotic surgeon, he's defined the field. He also does virus research. He's just a great mind and a wonderful person. Then he recruited equally talented surgeons."

Rosen then turned his sights on Dr. Larry Kwak, head of MD Anderson's multiple myeloma and lymphoma program. Years before, the two had studied together at Northwestern.

"He's brilliant. He won the Korean government's equivalent of the Nobel Prize," Rosen said. "Larry came. With Larry's arrival, suddenly there is recognition in that domain."

Rosen recruited Dr. Guido Marcucci, a national figure in the treatment of leukemia, and Dr. Ravi Salgia of the University of Chicago, who was brought in to head City of Hope's department of medical oncology.

Rosen said, "Now people call us. They're leaving tenure-track positions where they have security to come to an institution where we give three-year rolling contracts. That is because they feel like the resources are so remarkable and the environment so supportive that they will thrive."

Both T.J. Gernon and Erminia Massarelli, the two physicians on the front lines of Fred Claire's treatment, were part of City of Hope's remarkable influx of talent. Massarelli, the protégé of Jim Allison at MD Anderson, was recruited to expand the City of Hope program for treating head and neck cancers, continue her immunotherapy research, and initiate clinical trials. She found that her new professional home was the equal of more well-known places.

"If you go by reputation of the best cancer hospitals, MD Anderson still ranks first," she said. "MD Anderson is like an empire with twenty thousand employees and two thousand oncologists. It's huge. City of Hope is not like this, of course, but it's amazing. How many oncologists? Not even three hundred. But then when you see the number of trials we have opened and the opportunities for the patients, they are equivalent to MD Anderson."

She was just as impressed by the City of Hope culture: "We're not hiring less-famous people than MD Anderson. We're attracting highly qualified physicians with wonderful track records. In 2018, Dr. Mike Caligiuri [a nationally known researcher and clinician in the field of blood diseases] came in as president. But what is unbelievable is that I can talk to Caligiuri. I can call him. I can send him a message. Dr. Rosen, oh my gosh, he answers you immediately. Coming from a huge institution, it was a very competitive place. Here the stress level is less. We're very close to each other. There is no distance. There are no layers. Every physician feels appreciated as much as the others. I don't see anybody unhappy here."

And no City of Hope clinician or researcher, no matter what their previous achievements, would work alone. Rosen institutionalized that collegiality by creating the "tumor boards," which are multidisciplinary teams that collaborate in the cases of each patient.

"As an example, I may be the most knowledgeable in my given area, but we work as a team," Rosen said in a 2019 interview. He pulled up a cell phone photograph showing himself in a room full of scientists and physicians who had gathered to discuss a case. "This is from yesterday morning," he said. "We are all together, with the microscopes, with the patient data, with the photographs—pathologists, dermatologists, medical oncologists, social workers—discussing what is the best approach for that patient. In ninety-nine percent of the other places, you're seeing one doctor who is giving their opinion. It may be right most of the time, but not always. There is a lot of experience in that room. And there is great camaraderie within the disease teams."

Attracting the world's finest clinicians and researchers to City of Hope was the most glamorous aspect of the institution's transformation. But equally crucial was the construction of an operating system to capitalize on its unique advantages. For example, there were few medical centers in the world where world-class researchers worked just a few hundred yards from patients who might benefit from their discoveries. The City of Hope shorthand was "bench to bedside."

Ashley Baker Lee again: "City of Hope had the ability to work on a new therapy or drugs in the preclinical phases, on the bench as it were, actually see them get approved by the Food and Drug Administration, and activate clinical trials for patients here. That, to me, really is the secret sauce of City of Hope. It's nimble enough to move quickly. Most other organizations are so bureaucratic. The infrastructure required for all of this is just too much, and they end up doing a lot of outsourcing. They often lose sight of the fact that, at the end of the day, it's about the patient."

Since her arrival in Duarte in 2012, Baker Lee had been responsible for deciphering the fog of regulation and bureaucracy to speed the delivery of new therapies to desperate patients. For her, the job was intensely personal. She lost both parents and a husband to cancer and is a survivor of the disease herself.

"To me it's all about speed," she said. "I'm not going to sit there in front of a patient and say, 'Gee, I'm sorry we couldn't get our act together, so we couldn't open this therapy for you.' Unless it's touched you, you really don't realize that 'wait' is a four-letter word."

At most other cancer centers, where new therapies are concerned, testing and red tape are necessary to meet regulatory requirements, and the development of clinical trial protocols are needed to be done elsewhere.

"That causes a time delay because you're coordinating with a lot of vendors," Baker Lee said. "At City of Hope, you can just walk across the hall and start talking about it. All of these services are available to the faculty. That's what cuts down on the time."

When Rosen arrived at City of Hope, it typically took more than a year for new clinical trials to be activated for patients.

"What pharmaceutical company is going to want to work with you if your activation time is a year?" Rosen said. "To them, every week costs them money. I told Ashley that the highest priority is to get the activation time down to three months, and she did it. She put together a workflow which would allow many different components to be done simultaneously. We met all the National Cancer Institute requirements, but in a very expedited manner. The record for one of my patients is that we initiated a trial in six weeks. So, now every pharmaceutical company wants to work with us. We have probably the most rapid activation time of any academic center. It's eighty-two days—almost unheard of."

By 2019, more than one thousand City of Hope patients were part of clinical trials, double the number of five years before. Federal grants to City of Hope researchers, another telling metric, had also doubled during the same period. More and more patients from around the world were coming to Duarte, and hospital beds were almost always full.

"When you bring on the most talented clinicians and clinical investigators and thought leaders in the field, everyone wants to send their patients to them," Rosen said.

In 2019, *U.S. News and World Report* listed City of Hope as the eleventh best cancer center in the nation for adults, up ten places from the previous year. It was the top-rated cancer center in the western United States.

"We would have told you fifteen years ago that we were the best-kept secret in the San Gabriel Valley," Robert Stone said in 2019. "That's changing very quickly. The growth over just the last five years has been tremendous. It allows us to serve more and more people. I'm not at all concerned about what the public knowledge is of City of Hope. More than enough people know what we do. That narrative has shifted dramatically over the last few years."

Stone continued: "Twenty-three years ago, when I joined City of Hope, we were primarily a hospital that did some science. Today, I would tell you that we're an organization that does cutting-edge scientific work and also provides great care. We understand that speed matters to cancer patients waiting for the next breakthrough. The resulting discoveries and the reputations of the scientists, doctors, and staff who work here, the partnerships that we've made with likeminded organizations, and the impact our research has had on people around the globe have spread the news. If you are in the cancer world, you know who we are today."

Robert Stone met Fred Claire soon after Fred arrived at City of Hope with a dire diagnosis and a desire to help.

"I've gotten to know Fred, and I found him to be what you would expect—thoughtful, earnest, brave, courageous," Stone said. "Wanting not only to go through his journey but also help others and make a difference to increasingly larger audiences. He has always struck me as somebody who is focused more on helping people through that journey than he is about looking inward and asking how he is going to take that journey himself. He recognizes that he has a unique capacity for bringing hope to others and make a difference to increasingly larger audiences.

"I've been here twenty-three years, and one of the great attributes of the people I've been fortunate enough to run across over that time is that they don't necessarily come into it wanting to shine the light on themselves. I know a lot of great cancer centers, great physicians, and great researchers who I wouldn't say the same thing about. For us, it's about helping individuals, but I'm grateful Fred wants to shine the light."

The former baseball executive would indeed become one of the medical center's most ardent and articulate advocates.

At the same time, in the course of a three-year medical journey at the institution, the cases of few other patients would prove as challenging, requiring the expertise and commitment of a broad array of City of Hope doctors, researchers, nurses, and therapists. By the winter of 2017, there was no better place to give Fred his last best chance of survival.

7

DESTINY INTERVENES

The sound was unlike anything heard before in the quarter century that baseball had been played at Dodger Stadium. What began as a relative murmur grew into a cacophonous roar as fifty-six thousand people, most of them wearing blue, realized what was happening: Kirk Gibson was hobbling toward home plate.

It was October 15, 1988, and a typically gorgeous Southern California night. In the first game of the World Series, the visiting and heavily favored Oakland A's led 4–3 in the bottom half of the ninth inning. The Dodgers were down to their final out when Gibson emerged from the dugout. The team's star slugger and emotional leader was so diminished by injuries to both legs that he was incapable of participating in the ceremonial pregame introductions. Yet here he was, in the ninth, pausing at the on-deck circle to rub down his brown bat with a sticky rag. He took a couple of tentative and clearly painful practice swings. Then Gibson limped toward the home plate and destiny, covered over by the din.

What happened next would go down as one of the most memorable moments in the history of baseball, and in the long history of a franchise that had begun in Brooklyn 105 years before. The drama and magnitude of Kirk Gibson's moment were such that they overshadowed the events of the two previous weeks, which, in so many ways, were just as unlikely, just as remarkable.

•◆•

Given the odds against the Dodgers, Gibson should never have had the chance to become a World Series legend. To get to the Fall Classic, the Dodgers had to overcome their National League rivals, the New York Mets, who had outscored them 49–14 in eleven regular season meetings.

The Dodgers acquitted themselves well at Dodger Stadium in the first two games of the 1988 National League Championship Series, winning one. But the next three games would take place in the autumn madness that is playoff baseball in New York.

"In Shea Stadium and New York in big games, it was almost as if the stadium kind of moved," Fred Claire recalled years later. "It literally rocked and rolled, so there was that type of atmosphere. The other thing about that series was the absolute feeling of the intensity. The Mets had dominated us, and now, with all we had done before in that season, it wouldn't mean anything unless we overcame this incredible obstacle."

Game Three at Shea Stadium in Queens began well for the visitors, who clung to a one-run lead in the eighth inning. To protect it, the Dodgers turned to their ace reliever, Jay Howell. But as Howell battled his first hitter, Mets manager Davey Johnson unexpectedly climbed from the dugout and approached the home plate umpire, who in turn convened a historic conclave at the pitcher's mound. It was joined by Dodger players, manager Tommy Lasorda, and third-base umpire Harry Wendelstedt, the chief of the umpiring crew. It was Wendelstedt who took Howell's glove, poked and prodded, and eventually discovered a sticky, forbidden substance called pine tar. When applied, it enabled a pitcher to have a firmer grip and better control.

"It was late in the year when it's cooling off, and you have a pitch that requires a good grip, like a breaking ball. That was my out pitch," Howell recalled in 2019. "I figured a little pine tar might help. So, Johnson comes out, and it's a big deal."

Wendelstedt rubbed his fingers together as if to confirm the crime, and then, as the New York crowd roared, raised his right fist, signifying that Howell had been ejected from the game. The veteran umpire marched the glove to the first-row seat of Bart Giamatti, the Commissioner of Baseball, another act of dramatic damnation.

"Can you believe this?" television announcer Al Michaels said. "This has never happened to my knowledge in the postseason."

"Dodgers Cheat! Dodgers Cheat! Dodgers Cheat!" The Shea Stadium chant grew louder, washing over Fred and Sheryl Claire as they sat with Dodger owner Peter O'Malley and his family in the visiting team box near the playing field. The Claires would never forget the humiliation of that moment.

"I have seldom been so upset in my entire life as I sat there with my wife, Sheryl—and Peter O'Malley and his wife, Annette, and O'Malley's sister, Terry Seidler—watching this scene play out," Fred Claire wrote in his memoir. "At that point, I wasn't sure what Wendelstedt had discovered on Jay's glove, but my anger increased with every passing moment. Quite frankly, I felt terrible for Peter and his family to be sitting there, after all of their heartfelt efforts, hearing fans yell, 'Dodgers Cheat!'"

The Dodgers also collapsed that day on the field, eventually losing 8-4. After the game, Claire stormed into the office of Lasorda, insisting they be joined by Howell and pitching coach Ron Perranoski.

"I don't know what the hell happened out there today, but I have only one thing to say," Claire told them. "No matter what happened or what the background was, the only thing we say to the National League office is the absolute truth. Anything other than that is unacceptable to me. We are all in this situation together, and we will face it together."

To *Los Angeles Times* sports columnist Bill Plaschke, it was one of Claire's finest moments: emblematic of his character.

"Today, Jay Howell would have hid behind his agent or attorneys, and it would have been a national scandal," Plaschke said in 2019. "Fred made him talk about what he did, admit what he did, so they could put it behind them, and this was in the middle of the postseason. That's toughness."

In the next game, Game Four, the Dodgers trailed 4-2 in the ninth inning and faced Mets pitching star Dwight "Doc" Gooden. Los Angeles seemed almost certain to fall into a 3-1 series deficit from which few teams ever recover.

Destiny intervened.

How else could you explain the ninth-inning plate appearance of John Shelby, the Dodger's journeyman outfielder known for chasing down fly balls and, at times, chasing pitches that were well out of the strike zone?

"Shelby would not walk in a pedestrian zone," Dodger third-base coach Joey Amalfitano told writer K.P. Wee decades later. "He walked him! That happened almost thirty years ago, but I could still see Doc Gooden's eyes when he walked Shelby, like, 'What did I just do?'"

Mike Scioscia was up next. The veteran Dodger catcher and team leader was best known for his prowess behind the plate. That season, he had hit just three home runs.

Again, destiny intervened.

When Gooden grooved his first pitch, Scioscia pounced, lining it into the bullpen behind the right field fence to tie the score.

"It got so quiet when I hit that home run, I remember running and hearing my spikes hit the dirt," Scioscia recalled years later.

That was when the notion began to take hold in the Dodger dugout and beyond that this strange bunch of overachievers assembled by Fred Claire had the wind of fate at their backs. That sense grew even more pronounced that night as the deadlocked game entered the twelfth inning. Kirk Gibson had been feebly retired in five previous at-bats in the game, but his sixth trip to the plate in the twelfth foreshadowed what was to come. Gibson launched a towering solo home run to give his team a slender lead.

Then, if anything, the drama intensified. The Mets loaded the bases in the bottom of the inning. With two outs, and Howell, his best reliever, suspended because of the pine tar incident, Lasorda turned to Orel Hershiser, the Dodger ace starter who had pitched seven innings just the day before.

"I got suspended, and we were a player down, and it dawned on me over the years that I essentially put my team at risk," Howell recalled. "But the guys in the bullpen picked me up. And my absence led to what happened with Orel. I think about that today every time I see a starter come in from the bullpen in a World Series game. I think about Orel, The Bulldog. A big part of that team was one guy filling in for the other guy, the selflessness of that and everybody having your back. They had my back."

On Hershiser's third pitch, batter Kevin McReynolds lofted a soft blooper to center field that seemed destined to drop in front of Shelby, which would have delivered the pivotal win to New York. In another crucial moment of an earlier game of the series, Shelby could not make the catch on a very similar play.

"We ended up losing that game," Shelby remembered. "I wanted another chance. You never know if you're going to get it. When that ball was hit, my initial thought was that I've got a chance. I never thought about missing the ball again. My whole instinct was, 'You're going to make the catch. You're going to make the catch.'"

Shelby raced in and snatched the ball at his kneecaps for the final out.

"I gave a sigh of relief," Shelby said. "I mean, it was just excitement to know we had beat them. We knew we were up against a tough ball club. Just knowing that I helped seal the victory—it was just pure excitement. Every time we won a game it was a celebration, so it was another time to go in and celebrate."

"When you write the story of this game," Al Michaels asked his television audience, "where in the world do you begin?"

The teams split the next two contests, but Game Seven in Los Angeles was almost anticlimactic. With Hershiser at his dominant best, the Dodgers smothered the Mets, 6–0.

The newly crowned National League champions were now increasingly compared to another Mets team from a generation before. Until 1969, those Mets had been known mostly for their historic ineptitude. Then, that magical autumn, the Miracle Mets parlayed superior pitching and pixie dust into baseball legend, defeating the Baltimore Orioles to win the World Series. Nineteen years later, that same dust seemed to have settled onto the shoulders of the team from Los Angeles.

•◆•

Even with both teams at full strength, the Oakland Athletics would still have been heavily favored to win the 1988 World Series. The American League champions had won 104 games that season and were imposing just to look at, led by Jose Canseco and Mark McGwire—sluggers known as the Bash Brothers—two guys who had physiques of NFL linebackers.

"It was a mismatch, David versus Goliath," Dodger catcher Rick Dempsey remembered. "They had all those gorillas over there."

To compound matters, the long, emotional series against the Mets meant that Orel Hershiser would be unavailable to pitch in the crucial first game of the World Series.

"We were happy about that," Oakland general manager Sandy Alderson remembered years later. "Hershiser wouldn't be able to pitch three times."

Most importantly, the Dodgers would be without their

leader, probably for the entire series. Kirk Gibson had been injured against the Mets, and for most of Game One at Dodger Stadium he wasn't even in the dugout or in uniform, but sitting in the clubhouse in gym clothes with ice packs on both legs. Every inning, Lasorda came back from the dugout to check on him, asking, "How are you feeling, big boy?"

Each time a dejected Gibson put his thumb down.

"He was really suffering, and he couldn't do it," Lasorda told Arash Markazi, a writer for *Sports Illustrated*, years later. "If he had half a chance of doing it, he would have done it, but he said, 'I just can't do it. My leg is really hurting me.' So I figured that was it."

Reduced to following the game on a clubhouse television, Gibson watched as his replacement, Mickey Hatcher, hit a two-run homer in the first inning to give the Dodgers a short-lived lead. In the next inning, Jose Canseco's violent grand slam home run dented a television camera in center field. The Dodgers added a run in the sixth but trailed heading into the bottom of the ninth, where Dennis Eckersley, baseball's best relief pitcher, awaited them.

In the late innings, television cameras began to scan the Dodger dugout to catch sight of the moment Gibson finally appeared on the bench.

"There is no Gibson," Vin Scully finally told a national television audience. "The man who was the spearhead of the Dodgers' offense throughout the year, who saved them in the league championship series, will not see any action tonight for sure. He is not even in the dugout."

Gibson heard Scully on a locker room television.

"My ass," Gibson said.

A young clubhouse attendant named Mitch Poole was nearby, picking up towels.

"Go get my uniform, Mitch," Gibson said.

The player struggled into his Dodger whites and hobbled into an underground batting cage, where Poole placed balls on a batting tee. Gibson took five swings, trying to find a stance that would allow him to swing and not fall down.

"Mitch, go get Tommy," Gibson said.

Poole sprinted toward the dugout. Lasorda, plotting his ninth inning strategy, was at first irritated by the interruption.

"I said, 'Mitch, leave me alone, damn it! I'm trying to get this ninth inning set up,'" Lasorda told Markazi. "He said Kirk wanted to talk to me. I go there in the back, and Kirk has his uniform on. He says, 'I think I can hit for ya.'"

Eckersley had retired the first two Dodgers in the ninth, but walked a speedy pinch hitter named Mike Davis. Gibson was out of the dugout, bat in hand, before Davis had made it to first base.

"And look who's coming up," Scully said above the stadium crescendo. "All year long they looked to him to light the fire, and all year long he answered the demands until he was physically unable to start tonight with bad legs. With two outs, you talk about a roll of the dice. This is it. The Dodgers are trying to catch lightning in a bottle right now."

The noise continued to grow.

"The crowd ... I can never explain it," Lasorda remembered. "The emotion, the reaction of that crowd that night. I've been here a long time. I've never seen anything like that. I got goose bumps because of the reaction of the fans."

But Gibson's attempt, however valiant, seemed destined to fail. He waved weakly at Eckersley's first two pitches, fouling them off. He looked like a batter in no condition to compete.

"After he swung, he looked so feeble," Eckersley remembered years later. "I thought I was going to blow him away. I thought he was a lamb. I'm thinking I'm going to throw him a high fastball and he's done."

Many Dodgers silently thought the same thing.

"It was terrible. Just terrible," Hershiser recalled. "We were in the dugout thinking he shouldn't have even tried to hit."

Gibson's soft tapper, hit foul down the first base line, was no more encouraging. Eckersley then missed the strike zone with two pitches, evening the count at two balls and two strikes. Davis stole second base on the next pitch, also a ball.

"When Mike Davis finally got to second base, I thought, 'Just dink it over the shortstop. Just score him and tie it up,'" Gibson told *Sports Illustrated*. "That's really all I was thinking at the time. I was just thinking about keeping the inning going."

But another thought soon entered Gibson's mind. He remembered super scout Mel Didier's pregame report on the Oakland pitchers.

"After I was done talking to the team about each guy, I turned, and all the left-handed hitters were sitting on the floor in the dressing room," Didier later told *Sports Illustrated*. "There was Kirk and Scioscia and Mike Davis and all the left-handed guys, and I pointed to them and said, 'Now remember, if you're up in the ninth inning and we're down or it's tied and you get to 3-and-2 against Eckersley—partner, sure as I'm standing here breathing, you're going to see a 3-2 backdoor slider.'"

He referred to a breaking pitch designed to catch the outer edge of home plate against a left-handed hitter.

Gibson stepped out of the batter's box and repeated Didier's words to himself: "Partner, sure as I'm standing here breathing . . . "

He leaned over the plate in anticipation, watching as, sure enough, Eckersley's backdoor slider spun toward him. Using nothing but his arms, Gibson launched the pitch into the California night. Even Vin Scully seemed momentarily taken aback.

"High fly ball into right field," Scully yelled finally. "She is gone."

Scully was silent for minutes after that, letting the sights and sounds of history play out on the field below him. Gibson limped around the bases, pumping his fist, and somehow managed to touch home plate with the winning run as he was mobbed by his teammates. Euphoria poured down from the stands.

"In a year that has been so improbable, the impossible has happened," Scully said.

On radio, another legendary broadcaster, Jack Buck, put it this way: "I don't believe what I just saw."

Fred Claire watched from his box above the field. For him, there was nothing more to be done that night. He closed his briefcase.

"I left my box, as I had done after hundreds of games, and walked along the club level of Dodger Stadium, and there was nobody in the aisles," he remembered. "Everybody was still standing at their seats. I stopped by my office and then walked out the main entrance, and it seemed like there was nobody in the parking lot. I walked to my car and drove out of Dodger Stadium, and I was literally the only car driving in the lot. There was still such a roar behind me. It was almost like a *Twilight Zone* episode. It was so surreal. It was truly an unreal scene. I've never experienced anything like it."

It was just one game, of course . . . but it wasn't. Rarely in the history of baseball had a single playoff win been as exhilarating for the victors and as dispiriting for the team that lost. Destiny turned out to be a confounding foe for the A's. Canseco's grand slam was his only hit in what turned out to be a five-game series. Mark McGwire had only one hit himself.

The Dodgers' leading hitter for the series was Mickey Hatcher, the first player Fred Claire had acquired on his second day as general manager. Were it not for Claire's offer of a contract, Hatcher, who had just been released by the Twins, likely would have been out of the game. Had it not been for Gibson's injury, Hatcher would have spent most of the World Series on the bench. Destiny intervened.

"I was on my way out of baseball, and Fred Claire was my last hope," Hatcher recalled decades later. "He revived me and got me a couple of more years in the game. He definitely was a big part of how my career ended: just a super person who believed in me and who gave me another shot and gave me a chance to win a World Series."

Hatcher might have been the Most Valuable Player of the World Series had it not been for Hershiser, who was virtually unhittable in the second game against the A's, another 6–0 blowout win for the Dodgers.

Hershiser was back on the mound for Game Five, with the Dodgers needing only one more win to take their place in history. Leading 5–2 with two out in the ninth, the A's were down to their last strike. Hershiser's fastball overpowered the A's hitter, Tony Phillips, popping into the glove of Rick Dempsey. Months before, in Fred Claire's office, as he lobbied for a chance to play, Dempsey had foretold the moment. He was behind the plate in the last game because of an injury to Mike Scioscia. Destiny intervened.

Dempsey was first to reach Hershiser in the joyous mob scene at the pitching mound.

"Like the 1969 Mets, it's the impossible dream revisited," Vin Scully told his television audience.

In the champagne-drenched locker room, Peter O'Malley was presented with the World Series trophy as Fred Claire and Tommy Lasorda looked on.

"For two years we suffered a great deal," Lasorda told announcer Bob Costas. "And now the Dodgers are back on top. We are the champions of baseball. They never quit believing in themselves. They have to be an influence on everybody in the world, because it shows you what someone can do when they really want something bad enough"

Costas turned to Claire. The Dodger general manager had been anticipating this moment for weeks, thinking about what he would say.

"In your first full season as general manager, what a dream come true," Costas said.

Claire's hair and shirt were soaked in champagne. His voice was hoarse.

"I give the credit to the players, to Tommy, to the staff, to every member of the Dodger organization because in this room tonight, I feel the presence of all those people," Claire said. "Our scouts, our minor league people, everyone who has contributed to the Dodgers past and present, they are with us tonight. We accept this on their behalf."

But Claire himself was hardly forgotten in the bedlam.

"Fred Claire just put an outstanding ball club on the field,"

Orel Hershiser told Costas during the celebration. "He went into the free-agent market and got us some big players. You've got to give that man a lot of credit also."

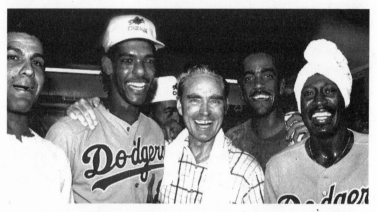

Fred celebrated with (from left) Mario Soto, Ramon Martinez, Gilberto Reyes, and Alfredo Griffin after the Dodgers clinched the National League West Division title in 1988.

A few minutes later, Dempsey made good on the promise he made to the general manager in Claire's office months before. The catcher reached into the back pocket of his uniform pants and pulled out the baseball from the final pitch.

"Fred, this belongs to you," Dempsey said.

Nearly three decades later, Bob Costas also recalled that night.

"On the field, the Dodgers were led by Tommy Lasorda—one of baseball's most colorful and bombastic characters of that, or any era," Costas wrote in *Shared*, Rich Kee's book that was a gift to the former general manager when he needed it most. "Meanwhile, the front office was headed by Fred Claire. As reserved a public figure as one could imagine. Without fanfare, Fred went about his duties—putting together the best team he could for Lasorda to manage and inspire."

Costas continued, "I'll always remember conducting the postgame interviews following the Dodgers unforgettable and emotional victory over the favored Oakland A's in the 1988 World Series. The clubhouse was jubilant. Lasorda was exultant. And there stood Fred Claire, beaming with pride, but deflecting almost all the credit to the champagne-soaked guys in uniform. In his own unassuming way, he was enjoying the pinnacle of an admirable baseball career. But doing it in a way that was true to himself . . . and the record speaks for itself. Fred is an accomplished baseball man. And in many moments, but especially at that one, I admired his integrity and demeanor."

· ◆ ·

In April 2017, with Fred's prognosis so dire, he and Sheryl invited Bill Plaschke to their Pasadena home for an interview. The *Los Angeles Times* columnist found Claire physically weakened by his cancer fight, but emotionally unbowed.

In his column that was published a few days later, Plaschke recalled the days when the scandal surrounding the firing of Al Campanis had plunged the Dodgers into darkness.

"In two short seasons, he built the Dodgers' sixth World Series championship team in the history of the legendary franchise, paved the way for Tommy Lasorda's election to the Hall of Fame, and helped create the greatest singular baseball moment in Los Angeles Dodgers history.

"His name is Fred Claire, and today, at age eighty-one, as he fights the ravages of jaw and neck cancer from the privacy of his Pasadena home, he is fine with the shadows.

"He has all he needs, and he knows right where it is.

"There's a championship banner down there at Dodger Stadium that says '1988,'" he says, his eyes welling. "That is enough."

In an interview two years later, Plaschke put it this way: "1988 secured Fred's spot as one of the all-time Dodger greats. Look, he achieved something that hasn't been done again in what, thirty years. He belongs in the pantheon with Koufax, Drysdale, Newcombe, Jackie Robinson, Lasorda, Vin Scully, all of them. He deserves that as much as any of the others."

8

HOW DO YOU EXPLAIN THAT?

J ust a few years before, perhaps even a few months before, Fred Claire's only remaining option would have been palliative care. When the cancer returned in early 2017, doctors would have attempted to manage the symptoms of advanced squamous cell carcinoma and mitigate the pain of what would have been an agonizing end. But that's all they could have done.

"It would have been a long, painful journey," said Massarelli, Claire's oncologist at City of Hope. "If nothing works in the end, you're just controlling the pain. Because the cancer had not spread, it would have been cancer in that one area for a long time, a year or longer, with worsening quality of life. The cancer would have eventually killed him. My gosh, he would have been in unbelievable pain."

That was the terrible reality confronted by Fred and Sheryl

Claire after Dr. Gernon found a lump in Fred's neck during that shattering appointment on February 21, 2017. Scans and a biopsy quickly confirmed the worst, multiple tumors in his neck and throat area. In the weeks to come, Fred could feel the tumors growing. The pain also returned.

"It looked like it was the end of the road," he said.

On March 6, 2017, the Claires made the familiar drive from their home in Pasadena to City of Hope for an afternoon appointment with Massarelli. She discussed palliative care. But as of just a few weeks before, she said, there might be another option for Fred at City of Hope.

She described a new clinical trial sponsored by pharmaceutical giant Bristol-Myers Squibb that was being conducted at major cancer centers across the nation. City of Hope was one of them. Massarelli was the lead clinician and investigator.

That day in her office, the oncologist explained how immunotherapy had begun to revolutionize cancer treatment. Until just a few years before, the human immune system had been mysteriously neutralized in the fight against cancer. But recent breakthroughs in cancer research had shown that drugs called "checkpoint inhibitors" could be stunningly effective at unleashing the immune system in the battle against the disease.

The new trial explored whether two checkpoint inhibitors, administered to a patient simultaneously, would be more effective in combating cancer than just one. It was a blind trial, Massarelli said, meaning that randomly selected patients would receive two drugs, while others would get one checkpoint inhibitor and a placebo. No one involved in the trial would know who was getting what.

In the last few years, going back to her time working with

Nobel Prize-winning researcher James Allison at MD Anderson in Houston, Massarelli had seen immunotherapy work wonders, helping patients who were only weeks from death achieve long remissions. But she was careful not to give the Claires false hope. Studies showed that immunotherapy was effective in only about one in five cases. What's more, she said, when the immune system was unleashed, it could attack healthy tissue as well as cancer cells, raising the possibility of dangerous and agonizing side effects.

Still, the oncologist said, "If this were my father, this is what I would recommend."

The Claires did not hesitate. After two terrible weeks, they had been offered a glimmer of hope.

"Our backs were against the wall," Sheryl Claire remembered. "We had no other options. We saw this as a wonderful opportunity that would not have been available to us even a short time before."

On March 27, Fred sat down in a City of Hope infusion room for the first of what would be seven intravenous immunotherapy treatments that would be administered every other week. In typical cases, it takes about two months for checkpoint inhibitors to stoke up the immune system, but within just a few weeks of his first treatment, Fred began to notice that the pain in his neck was subsiding. The area around the tumors had softened to the touch. He could turn his head with greater ease. Something was happening.

"T.J. Gernon said that would not happen unless the drugs were working," Sheryl said. "But it was so new, we didn't want to get ahead of ourselves. We were guinea pigs."

The results of his first scan, on May 3, were also hopeful. The tumors had not grown in the two months since the treatment.

"The cancer was stable," Massarelli recalled. "This was good."

A month later, on the evening of June 10, she and Dr. Forman were among the guests of the Claires at Dodger Stadium. On that remarkable night for Fred and his family, the City of Hope physicians witnessed healing of a very different sort.

•◆•

Fred Claire's thirty years in Dodger blue ended nineteen years before, almost to the day, on Father's Day, June 21, 1998. That weekend, he and Sheryl were in Denver for the last game of a road trip. Early on that Sunday, Fred called his daughter, Jennifer, to wish her a happy birthday. A few minutes later, a reporter called Fred with the news that Al Campanis had died.

"My life was inextricably tied to his," Claire wrote later in his memoir. "I had become the Dodger general manager only because of Al's unfortunate remarks on *Nightline* in 1987 that had cost him his job. But beyond the personal considerations, I felt the loss of one of the steadiest and oldest links to the Brooklyn years. I thought of this tragic news as the passing of an era. How ironic, considering that my career as a Dodger executive would pass as well in a few hours."

After the championship season in 1988, the Dodgers had returned to the playoffs on only two other occasions over the next decade, losing in the first round both times.

"I regretted it every year that we didn't win, but I always tried to use the experience to make us better the next year," Claire recalled.

Tommy Lasorda had retired in 1996 after suffering a heart

attack. By the summer of 1998, the Dodgers were limping along, well out of first place. But it wasn't the performance of the team that most threatened Claire's long tenure.

The previous March, the universe of the Los Angeles Dodgers had been turned upside down—Peter O'Malley had sold the team to media mogul Rupert Murdoch and his Fox Group. Though O'Malley briefly stayed on in a figurehead position, previously unthinkable occurrences began to take place within the organization.

The most striking came in May, when Dodger superstar catcher Mike Piazza was traded to the Florida Marlins by the team's new leadership—without the knowledge of Fred Claire. The team's new president, Bob Graziano, told Claire about the trade during a game at Dodger Stadium, saying it needed to be announced afterwards.

Claire replied that there would be two announcements: the trade and his own resignation.

"This is not the way the Dodgers operate," a furious Claire told Graziano. "You don't need a general manager if trades are being made without his involvement."

It became even messier from there. The transaction could not be announced after all, because the player the Dodgers were to acquire for Piazza, Gary Sheffield, had a "no-trade" clause in his contract. That had yet to be sorted out, which Claire and any other general manager would have known.

"The people making this trade had no clue," Claire recalled.

Yet he decided to stay on to help the organization he loved sort through its issues.

"I wasn't going to walk away and leave this mess of a trade, even though I hadn't been involved," Claire said years later.

Then came Father's Day. That day in Denver, not long after

learning of Campanis' death, Claire received a call and was told to be at Dodger Stadium that night for a meeting with Graziano as soon as the team returned to Los Angeles.

"A Sunday night meeting after a road trip was highly unusual and sounded awfully important, but I didn't push for details," Claire wrote. "Still, I couldn't get it out of my mind. The team was struggling. The media was questioning the team's direction under the ownership of Rupert Murdoch's Fox Group, and the fans were restless and unhappy after the Piazza trade. In that time of turmoil, anything was possible.

"And I knew that the Fox people were unhappy with me because when the Piazza trade ultimately went through, I talked publicly about how it had come about and how I had felt about it."

The Sunday night meeting took place in what had once been Peter O'Malley's office, where Claire had spent countless hours as the trusted and longtime executive who had worked so closely with the Dodger owner. O'Malley, in fact, sat in on what would be a very different gathering, one in which Graziano did most of the talking. He told Claire that manager Bill Russell would be fired.

"Then the other shoe hit the floor with a thud that shook my very being," Claire recalled.

He, too, was being let go, Graziano told him. Tommy Lasorda would be named the interim general manager.

"At age sixty-two, after a lifetime of steady employment in an unsteady field, I had just been fired for the first time," Claire wrote. "That I had lasted so long didn't lessen the blow, ease the pain or soften my resolve to maintain my dignity and my convictions."

That night, Claire wanted it made known that he had been terminated.

"They were not going to say Fred Claire quit," he remembered. Claire called his wife after the meeting.

"Are you sitting down?" he said. "I've just been fired. Would you come to Dodger Stadium and pick me up? We're going home."

"I'll be right there, sweets," she said.

The next day, Fred and Sheryl returned to Dodger Stadium to clean out his office. For nineteen years after that, she would never return. Fred went back on only a couple of occasions at the request of friends, including an invitation from Dodger great Maury Wills, which came after the team had been sold again, this time to businessman Frank McCourt.

Years later, Claire said he was never bitter about the way his years with the Dodgers ended. "I knew I had given the Dodgers the best I had each and every day," he recalled in 2019.

As much as anyone, Claire also knew the realities of professional sports. He himself had released many players over his time as general manager. What was more difficult to reconcile were the memories of a family-owned sports franchise that had placed such a premium on continuity and loyalty—values clearly not part of the corporate philosophy of the new ownership.

Claire's career was just one prominent example of the old ways. He had earned the trust and respect of Peter O'Malley over many years, which went far to explain the owner's decision after the 1987 season to retain Claire as general manager. With the new ownership, a much different calculus would clearly be brought to bear.

For Claire, cherished relationships built over three decades were altered by the way his Dodger days came to an end. He remained cordial with Peter O'Malley, but their friendship would be more distant. After Lasorda succeeded Claire as general manager, tension lingered between the two men for years.

Their friendship dated to 1969, when Claire was still a sportswriter and Lasorda a minor league manager. That was when the manager had actually put Claire into a spring training game as a shortstop for his Spokane team, replacing Bobby Valentine, who went on to become a successful major league manager himself.

"Fred and I are as close as brothers," Lasorda had been fond of saying.

"It was a generally good relationship, even after I became general manager at a time when Tommy already was a veteran manager with hopes of becoming a GM himself one day," Claire said later. "The GM-manager relationship is never easy, but Tommy and I worked well together in those roles for a decade because we both had a burning desire to see the Dodgers succeed."

The two men would also be forever linked by the magic of 1988. But after Claire's firing a decade later, and until 2017, their relationship was strained and Fred blamed himself.

"I made comments about changes in the coaching staff after I was fired that shouldn't have been made," he said in 2019. "I was no longer there. It wasn't my place to comment."

•—◆—•

By 2017, the Dodgers had been to the playoffs for four straight years, and with a new generation of stars like slugger Cody Bellinger and pitching ace Clayton Kershaw, the team seemed positioned to win its first championship since 1988. Amid the growing buzz in Los Angeles, Bill Plaschke, the *Los Angeles Times* sports columnist, remembered another Dodger legend who had disappeared from the public eye: "Everyone was talking about the great new Dodger era and all the division championships like it had never been done before. And I thought, 'Wait a minute. The general manager of the last World Series champion is right down the street and you've forgotten all about him.' He had never been truly honored at Dodger Stadium and that was a shame. I didn't want this great man and his great accomplishments to be forgotten."

That was what inspired Plaschke's visit to the Pasadena home of Fred and Sheryl Claire in April 2017, and the newspaper column that appeared a few days later.

"You may barely remember him," he wrote. "His contributions have never been publicly honored. He has never thrown out a first pitch. His face has never been shown on a video board. He was ushered away from [Dodger Stadium] twenty years ago and has rarely returned since.

"But the echoes of [the stadium] will always include him, because Dodger history was forever changed by him. In a dramatic reversal unmatched in franchise lore, the former sportswriter weaved a classic comeback tale that stabilized a franchise, immortalized a manager, and helped turn lost souls into champions."

Plaschke's words resonated throughout the Dodger nation and in the front office of the team itself. A few days after the column was published, Fred Claire got a call from Lon Rosen, the team's executive vice president and chief marketing officer.

"Plaschke nailed us," Rosen told Claire. "He's right. This is long overdue."

He invited Claire to throw out the ceremonial first pitch on June 10 before the Dodger game against Cincinnati.

"When was the last time you threw a baseball?" Sheryl asked her husband when she heard.

"Love, I've been throwing a baseball all my life," Fred said.

"Yes, but how long has it been?"

"About twenty years," Fred said.

A few days later, his wife came home with two new baseball gloves and a ball. For weeks leading up to the big night, as Fred continued his last-ditch cancer treatment, the couple played catch in the driveway of their home.

• ◆ •

Not coincidentally, June 10 was also the date of the Dodgers' annual Oldtimers Game. Orel Hershiser was back in uniform that night, with Mickey Hatcher and past team greats like Ron Cey, Steve Garvey, Fernando Valenzuela, Don Newcombe, and Joe Torre, a former manager of the team. Before the gates were opened to the fans, Fred Claire stepped onto the field in a dark dress shirt and khaki pants for an easy, laugh-filled reunion with people who had been at the heart of his professional life for three decades. It was as if Claire had never been away. Current players also waited their turn to shake the hand of the man who was quietly such a part of Dodger lore, and the architect of the team's last championship.

At one point, a Dodger employee handed Claire a package that contained the familiar white jersey with blue trim. When Claire unfolded it, he saw his name on the back over the number 88. He was initially reluctant to put it on.

"I always felt that jerseys were earned by the players," he recalled. "I didn't play the game. They played the game. I always had total respect for that."

But Claire made an exception that night. He put the jersey on and stood on the third base line for the National Anthem, next to Sheryl and his daughters, Jennifer and Kim, his young granddaughter, Tyler, and Dodger manager, Dave Roberts.

Then came something Claire was not expecting.

"A few of us knew ahead of time what was going to happen," said Rich Kee, Claire's close friend who was on the field to photograph the moment. "He did not. The announcer directed everyone's attention to the left field message board."

A video tribute began to play.

"There are moments in Dodger history that fans will never forget. We remember those moments thinking of the players on the field," the narrator said. "Sometimes it's worth remembering the people behind the scenes, the ones who put those players in a Dodger uniform.

"Would Jackie Robinson have taken the field as a Dodger without Branch Rickey? And would Kirk Gibson have hit one of the most historic home runs in baseball history without former general manager Fred Claire making the move to bring him to the team?"

The screen showed Claire and Lasorda, champagne soaked, holding the World Series trophy, and the two men posing with the trophy and President Ronald Reagan and his wife, Nancy.

The narrator recalled how Rick Dempsey had presented the general manager with the ball from the final pitch of the 1988 World Series, saying, "Fred, this belongs to you."

"Fred donated the ball to the Baseball Hall of Fame, where it is on display for all fans to see in an exhibit called Autumn Glory. Today, we're pleased to welcome back the man who brought autumn glory to Dodger Stadium."

Kee, capturing the moment with his camera, was standing a few feet away as Claire looked up at the screen.

"I started to see his face transform from surprise to deep emotion," Kee said. "He's a very proper person, and you don't see him show emotion in public. But I saw his face, and I was pretty sure I knew what he was thinking. 'This is my life. I've dedicated my life to my work, and I'm seeing it being played out on that screen.' He had never been shown that kind of appreciation. I think any guy standing there would have felt the same way. It was a cool thing."

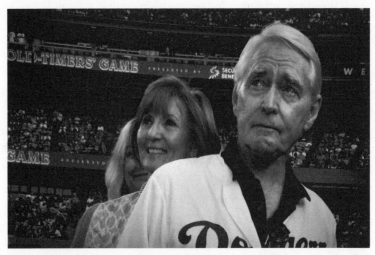

In a pregame ceremony at Dodger Stadium in 2017, Fred was surprised and emotional when the video board paid tribute to his thirty-year career with the Dodgers. Looking on with Fred are his wife, Sheryl, and daughter, Jennifer.

When the tribute was done, Claire was finally directed to take the pitcher's mound. He waved to a cheering crowd, then strode across the infield grass and toed the rubber before delivering a strike to Mickey Hatcher, who was waiting behind the plate.

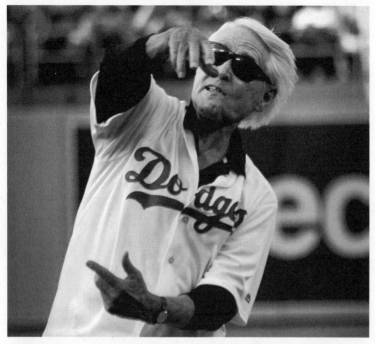

Fred had the honor of throwing out the ceremonial first pitch at Dodger Stadium in June 2017 and fired a strike with Mickey Hatcher on the receiving end.

As the game began, Claire, his family, and friends congregated in a stadium suite.

"It was up there that I checked the images in my camera, and I said, 'Fred I think I've just taken my best photograph from all my years at Dodger Stadium.' He looked at it—the picture that showed his eyes filling with tears as he watched the video—and he said, 'My goodness, Rich.' Given how personal it was, I didn't want to show the photo around without his approval. He said, 'Rich, emotions are human and photographs don't lie. Please feel free to use it.'"

But that night, the greatest healing took place out of the spotlight.

•◆•

Claire knew that Tommy Lasorda was likely to be at the ballpark for the Oldtimers event and hoped to make the most of an opportunity.

"I wanted to see resolution," Claire recalled. "I wanted Tommy to know how much I cared for him and how much his friendship of almost fifty years meant to me. I didn't want those distant feelings to be there, and I didn't know how much time I had left. If I didn't say that night what I wanted to say, I didn't know if I would have had the chance two months from then."

Early in the evening, as Claire and his daughters, Jennifer and Kim, walked through a stadium concourse, they saw Lasorda headed in their direction, riding a motorized scooter. His aide, Felipe Ruiz, was walking beside him. The former manager had recently been released from the hospital himself and looked frail.

"It's great to see you, Tommy," Claire said.

He leaned and put his arm around his friend.

"I love you, Tommy," Claire said softly.

"I love you, too," Lasorda replied.

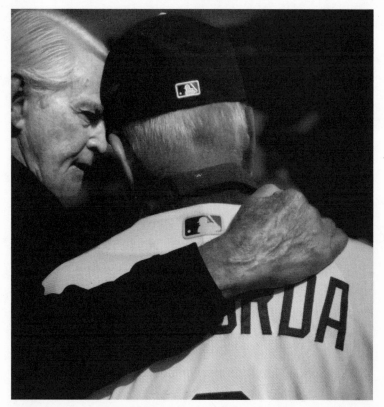

Hall of Fame manager Tommy Lasorda and Fred visited before the Oldtimers Game in 2017. The two first met in the spring of 1969 when Fred was a writer and Tommy was the manager of Spokane.

• ◆ •

A scan taken a few days later showed that, once again, Fred's tumors had not grown. Immunotherapy had seemed to battle his cancer to a stalemate. Nonetheless, the patient's health took another concerning turn. Fred suffered an attack of acute colitis, an inflammation of the colon. Tests also showed heart irregularities and problems with his adrenal glands. He was briefly hospitalized, and Massarelli prescribed high doses of steroids to combat the intestinal problem.

But the additional medications meant that Fred could no longer be a part of the clinical trial. His seventh immunotherapy infusion, administered on June 19, would be his last.

To the Claires, it seemed like another devastating setback.

"You're thinking to yourself, 'We're not getting the immuno-therapy. We've got colitis,'" Sheryl remembered. "It's just a bad break every time you turn around."

It was also natural to wonder if, without the treatments, the cancer would again be free to resume its deadly rampage. Massarelli was concerned as well; privately, though, the oncologist also saw reasons for hope.

The colitis was clearly a side effect of immunotherapy, but the seriousness of the attack also suggested to Massarelli that her patient had received both of the checkpoint inhibitors, not just one. There was no doubt that Claire's immune system had been successfully supercharged.

"There is a correlation between the side effects and response," Massarelli said. "It means that the immune system reacted really well, in the sense that it got overactive. Super active. Once you release those brakes, the immune system becomes crazy. It goes and kills the tumors but also affects the other organs."

Only time would tell what that meant in Fred Claire's battle for survival, but the Claires and Massarelli did not have to wait long for an answer. Fred underwent his next scan on July 24. The next day, the patient and his wife looked over Massarelli's shoulder as the results came up on her computer screen.

In previous scans, dots of fluorescent white represented the tumors. On July 25, the dots had vanished. Massarelli pointed to the places where they had been just the month before.

"How do you explain that?" Sheryl asked.

"It's a miracle," Massarelli replied.

Massarelli would never forget the moment.

"I have few occasions to give good news to patients, but with immunotherapy, it's a little more often," Massarelli said in 2019. "I'm always a little careful, but I said, 'This is fantastic. I think it's working.' The tests showed there was nothing in the neck. It was very exciting."

The joy was tempered by a stubborn reality. The cancer could return as quickly as it disappeared. In a treatment that was still so experimental, there was no track record upon which to base a prognosis.

"We didn't have a five-year study," Fred said. "We didn't have a three-year study. We *were* the study."

Massarelli encouraged the Claires to be both hopeful and cautious.

"He was symptom-free, and the scans were good. We were all happy," Massarelli said. "But there is always a feeling that, 'Okay, let's live day by day because we don't know if the cancer is going to come back.'"

But every scan in the months to come was also clean. The same was still true after six months, which Massarelli considered an important milestone.

"Really, that was my victory," Massarelli said. "That was as happy as I've been. With every scan, all of us are scared. But after six months, I saw the tumor was not back. Fred was lucky. I can tell you that he's been lucky to survive. I don't know what it is about him. I truly think that if people are very active, trust in life and trust in people, it affects their immune system. There are some endorphins that benefit very positive people. This could be one explanation why."

•◆•

The Claires eventually resumed their lives—the treks together across the golf course, regular visits to their vacation home in the desert, and weekly breakfasts with friends at Pie 'n Burger. But the miracle had changed them both.

"When people would ask, 'How are you, Fred?' I would say, 'I'm blessed,'" he said in 2019. "I didn't say that when I was in my seventies and healthy before cancer. I would say, 'I'm great.' But I knew what had happened. I was aware of the blessing that I had received. Immunotherapy is the only reason I'm here today. The treatment of cancer by cutting, burning, and poisoning is going to be surpassed, thank the Lord, by science and medicine, which is the whole theme of the City of Hope. That's really what we're talking about here, why we're trying to shine a light on all this."

Sheryl found herself living with a new urgency.

"None of us knows when the last day will come," she said. "You want to make the most of every day, do the right things, say the right things. If you want to tell a person you love them, don't wait. It just puts things in perspective."

"I was just a basket case," she continued. "I don't mind saying that. The thought of losing Fred, is just like . . . he's my world. And we've just been very fortunate that we're here at the City of Hope."

A day in the fall of 2019 brought another jolt of perspective. On a visit to City of Hope, they learned that of the four patients there on the same clinical trial, Fred was the only one to survive. He looked down when he heard. His eyes misted as he reached out to hug his wife.

9

FAMILY IS FAMILY

On August 14, 2017, a typically radiant Southern California morning, Fred and Sheryl Claire turned into the parking lot of Oakmont Country Club in Glendale, where they are longtime members and have spent some of their happiest days over the years.

That day, Charlie Hough, the famous knuckleball pitcher, arrived at the same time. After sharing a hug and while walking toward the clubhouse, Hough and Claire laughed about the old times, especially the day of Tommy Lasorda's dare in 1969, when Claire was still a sportswriter and Hough a minor league pitcher. Claire had suited up and played shortstop for Lasorda's Spokane team in a spring training practice game against Bakersfield. Lasorda also concocted a foot race between Claire and Hough that Claire won going away.

"Hough is so slow that if he raced a pregnant woman, he would come in third," Lasorda said at the time.

But those moments with Hough were just the beginning of a day of laughter and reminiscence. Dozens of old friends had also gathered at Oakmont for the first Fred Claire Celebrity Golf Classic benefitting City of Hope.

Many of the attendees had prominently worn Dodger blue— Orel Hershiser and Mickey Hatcher; Tim Leary and Steve Yeager; Reggie Smith and Hall of Fame slugger Eddie Murray; old-timers like Sweet Lou Johnson, Ron Fairly, Al Ferrara, and Tommy Davis. In fact, all five of the Los Angeles Dodgers' World Championship teams were represented, dating to the first one in 1959.

Terry Seidler, daughter of legendary Dodger owner Walter O'Malley and sister of Peter, wore a charm on her necklace from the 1955 World Series, the team's first and only World Championship of the Brooklyn era. The O'Malleys were much beloved in the Dodger realm, but none more so than Terry, a person of great warmth who epitomized the spirit of the organization. To the Claires, Terry Seidler's presence made the day at Oakmont even more special.

Ann Meyers Drysdale is a basketball Olympian and widow of Dodger great Don Drysdale. Her husband's Hall of Fame career had ended in 1969, the same year Fred Claire's time with the Dodgers began. Don Drysdale, who went on to a long career as a broadcaster, was one of two people in the world who called Claire "Freddie." His wife, Ann, was the other.

"I always refer to Don's teammates and friends the way he did," she said.

During Fred's cancer battle, Ann's supportive cards arrived every few weeks without fail. Perhaps some of her concern was based on her own heartbreaking experience with the disease, having lost her brother, UCLA basketball legend David Meyers, and her sister-in-law, Theresa Meyers, who had also been a patient at City of Hope.

"Being a part of the Dodger family—I mean, family is family," Meyers Drysdale said in 2019. "And I certainly have a lot of respect for the doctors and nurses at City of Hope and all the lives that they touch. Freddie's cancer is devastating, yet he's such a fighter, and it's amazing what the doctors have done. I just wanted to show appreciation and support. And all the people at that first golf tournament showed again the Dodger family supports one of their own."

But it wasn't just Fred's baseball family. Old friends like USC Heisman Trophy winner Mike Garrett and UCLA basketball coach Jim Harrick came, too. Former Dodger batboy Ben Hwang flew in from the Bay Area, and Ari Kaplan, his wife and children made the trip from Chicago.

In 1989, Kaplan had been a Caltech freshman with revolutionary ideas for the baseball world and the math to back it up.

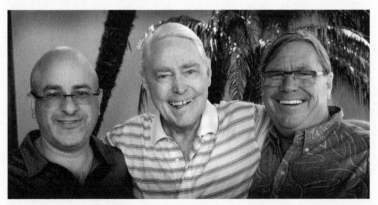

When Fred arrived for his first celebrity golf tournament to benefit City of Hope in 2017 at Oakmont Country Club, two of the first people to greet him were longtime friend Ari Kaplan (left) and Fred's son, Jeff (right).

"I had done a research project on how you can better evaluate players," Kaplan recalled in 2020. "I showed that a lot of the statistics that the press and the public were using—batting average, earned run average, wins, losses, and saves—were not always the best indicator of a player's performance. But instead of just complaining about it, I came up with my own approach, my own metrics. I started getting media attention from the *Los Angeles Times*, the *Today* show, CNN."

One day, when Kaplan was sitting in his college dorm, there was a knock at his door.

"This was before cell phones," he said. "The person at my door said a gentleman claiming to be the general manager of the Dodgers, Fred Claire, wanted to talk to me. Sure enough."

Claire wondered if Kaplan had time to meet him at Dodger Stadium in the next few weeks.

"I'll be there in a few hours," Kaplan replied.

Claire accompanied the student to the dugout and introduced him to Dodger coaches and players, wanting to have the young man's ideas evaluated by those closest to the game.

"Here I am, talking to Eddie Murray," Kaplan remembered. "I was showing the players charts, and they actually understood it and bought into it immediately. I remember saying to one of the pitchers, 'You are so much better than your statistics, and here's why.' They loved it."

Claire immediately began to integrate Kaplan's work into Dodger evaluations. While still at Caltech, Kaplan went on to work for the Baltimore Orioles and become one of the earliest pioneers of the analytics movement that would revolutionize the game. After graduating, Kaplan worked for thirty years in front offices, leading analytics for a number of major league teams. But he never forgot the call to his dorm.

"Basically, Fred thought that what I was doing could poten-tially help him and change the way players are evaluated," Kaplan said. "That's just from him being humble and realizing that he could be better at what he was trying to do. I love that about him. He helped me, for sure, but that was a great example of who he is. He wants to succeed, but in an appropriate way. Ask questions. Be humble. Don't cover up what you don't know. Instead embrace it and try to get better. That was a huge life lesson for me."

Claire and Kaplan remained close friends. Years later, after Claire left the Dodgers, the two men became partners in one of the game's top analytics companies, Ariball. Claire sug-gested the name.

"Ari had put together the technical work, and I wanted him to receive the credit and acknowledgment," Claire said.

The meeting between the young Caltech student and the veteran baseball executive came full circle in 2019, thirty years after their first encounter, when Claire received one of the insti-tute's highest honors—selection as an Honorary Member of the Caltech Alumni Association. It was Kaplan, a past winner of the Caltech "Alumni of the Decade," who had made the nomination.

"When his cancer was diagnosed, Fred was teaching the first ever sports class at Caltech and always encouraging students to look at the sports world as a possible career path," Kaplan said. "He deserved the alumni award more than anyone I could imagine. Two of his students are now working for the Dodgers, and several others are involved in the business aspect of sports. I'm honored to be his friend."

"All those years ago, for him to reach out to a college student with no experience, when he was already working with Tommy Lasorda and people at the highest level. It was amazing," Kaplan continued. "But even in the year 2020, there are people who are looking to get into the game or people who are in the game, and he's always willing to give free mentorship or advice, to review a paper, to review a resume. It takes a toll in terms of time and energy, but that's his consistency. In the thirty-plus years I've known him, he always takes time to return calls and help people out. That's part of his essence."

A version of Kaplan's regard for Claire was shared by all of those who gathered at Oakmont on that beautiful August day. Every time Fred turned around, there was another hand to shake, another old story to relive.

"There was just such a feeling of love, togetherness, and support," Sheryl remembered. "The outpouring for Fred just permeated the air."

•◆•

To think that in late 2016, when Claire conceived of the tournament, there was a real question as to whether he would survive to see it through. A terrible prognosis had become even more dire when his cancer returned in February 2017.

"With the benefit of hindsight, the golf tournament was a very good thing for Fred," Sheryl remembered. "But I really struggled with it. It wasn't so much that I didn't want him to do the tournament. I honestly wasn't sure he was going to be *alive* to do the tournament. And if he had a short time to live, I couldn't help but wish he would spend that time with me, with his family and friends, and not be working so hard on the planning."

But not for a second, even in the darkest times, did Fred consider abandoning his project. Instead, it became a blessing and an all-consuming distraction.

"If I made a list of twenty things I needed to do on a certain day, anything related to cancer treatment wasn't on it," Fred recalled. "There was nothing I could do about that. I just had to show up for appointments and follow the instructions. And Sheryl did the driving and made sure I followed instructions and took my medications night and day. This was something I had some control over, where I could make a difference.

"I was obsessed. I don't say that was a good thing, but that's the way I approached it. This couldn't fail. This had to be good. My name and the City of Hope name would be on the tournament. It was the right cause. I was just driven to do everything I could to make it as good and successful as possible. Many say that I was consumed by my work in my Dodger days. There were certainly similarities to that and this tournament. So many pieces had to be put in place. No detail could be overlooked. I knew I just had to give everything I had to give."

He worked closely with City of Hope staff and put together a tournament advisory committee of trusted colleagues and friends from his Dodger days. They were people like Mike Fox, Bill Shumard, Rich Kee, Steve Brener, Jeff Fellenzer, Barry Turbow, Marsha Collier, Brandon Averill, Darryl Dunn, Kaplan, and current Dodger historian Mark Langill.

"Many of the people I called upon were prominent in their respective fields, but they gave their full support and were never too busy for a conference call or to do anything we might need for the tournament," Fred said.

It was Fred who personally reached out to the retired athletes and the other celebrity attendees. Rod Carew quickly accepted Claire's invitation to receive the tournament's Celebration of Life Award, a trophy that would bear Jackie Robinson's words: "A life is not important except in the impact it has on other lives."

Yet, as the day of the tournament approached, Claire's wife and friends again began to worry that he might not make it after all. He seemed on the verge of collapsing, not from the cancer but from exhaustion. Steroids prescribed to treat his colitis kept him from sleeping at night and made him even more driven during the day. Sheryl was so concerned that she contacted the couple's personal physician, Dr. Michael Mellman, and Dr. Massarelli. Mellman has been a close friend and personal physician of the Claires for decades, since the time he served as a doctor for the Dodgers, and he has collaborated with the City of Hope medical team.

"It was like Fred's hair was on fire," Sheryl remembered thinking as she reached out to the physicians, who eventually agreed to reduce the dosage.

"He was running out of gas," Rich Kee said.

But the exhaustion suddenly fell away on the morning of August 14.

"We had done the work, and now it was like Opening Day," Fred remembered of the tournament. "There was no stress. It was there to be enjoyed. Every moment was a treasure. Every handshake and hug a treasure."

It went off without a hitch, with live radio and television coverage of the event that raised more than $250,000 for cancer research at City of Hope and brought widespread exposure to the medical center.

The closing dinner was held in a packed Oakmont banquet room. In the back of Fred's mind, uncertain as he was about his future, he knew that the gathering might also be a farewell. Attendees represented aspects of his life that he cherished most: his wife and daughters; his son, Jeff, a professional videographer and producer, who captured the event on film. His older brother, Doug, who would pass away two years later, attended with his family. Former Dodger players and employees filled other banquet tables, along with colleagues and former students from his teaching days, as well as friends from his Rose Bowl affiliation and Pasadena civic involvement.

Dodger broadcasting legends Ross Porter and Jaime Jarrin served as emcees. Dr. Forman, Fred's esteemed friend from City of Hope, gave a short speech about medical advances and the spirit of compassion. He then joined Fred to present the Celebration of Life award to Carew, a heart transplant recipient who had lost his teenage daughter, Michelle, to leukemia. During his own brief remarks, Carew spoke of his gratitude for his extended life as a result of the transplant, and the importance of medical research.

But the high point of the evening came when Fred introduced his oncologist, Dr. Massarelli; surgeon, Dr. Gernon; nurse, Candy Young; occupational therapists, Mahjabeen Hashmi and Miranda Freeman; and patient advocate, Lupe Santana, who were seated together at a place of honor at the front of the room.

"Before that night, Fred didn't have a forum to show his appreciation for them," Rich Kee said. "That evening he had the chance to tell them directly, and in front of all of those people, what they meant, not only to him, but to so many others."

As he stood at the podium, Fred struggled to speak through

his emotions: "I have been blessed to be around a lot of great teams, but this is my all-time team. But this isn't just my team. This team has served so many others."

A reverent silence fell over the room, then the sound of loud and extended applause.

"There wasn't a dry eye," Kee said.

Later, when the banquet room had emptied, Fred and Sheryl sipped glasses of wine, reflecting on the day with two City of Hope staff members who had also worked so hard to make it a success, Ken Birkett and Julie Filkoff.

Before he and his wife headed home, Fred checked his tote bag, wanting to be sure he had the dozens of cards signed at the tournament by the former major leaguers and others. Each contained a message of support for a person who had desperately wanted to attend but could not. That person was Kevin Towers, formerly the general manager of the San Diego Padres and Arizona Diamondbacks, now Fred's teammate in a mutual battle for survival.

•◆•

They were baseball's odd couple. Fred Claire was the former sportswriter who had come up through the marketing and publicity departments of the Dodgers, while Towers had been a promising minor league pitcher, then a highly regarded scout when his playing career had been cut short by injury. Towers was in his mid-thirties when promoted to general manager of the San Diego Padres in 1995. Claire, then the general manager of the Dodgers, was twenty-six years his senior.

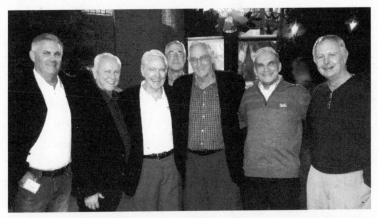

Great baseball friends (from left) Kevin Towers, Walt Jocketty, Fred, Cam Bonifay, Jerry Walker, Bruce Mano, and Terry Reynolds had a chance to visit and share memories at the 2015 baseball Winter Meetings.

The list of differences went on. Claire was famously reserved and proper, a person who kept his thoughts and feelings mostly to himself. Towers, known affectionately around the game as KT, was one of baseball's most gregarious and fun-loving characters.

Longtime baseball writer Bob Nightengale, who covered both men, recalled that when general managers gathered for annual meetings, parties afterward typically took place in Towers' hotel suite. He would be the one holding court, telling stories, filling the room with his laughter.

"Kevin was the life of every party; whereas, if Fred was there, he was standing in the back," Nightengale said. "If Fred had stories, he certainly would never share them. When you talk about general managers and try to name the two most unlikely to become close friends and hang out, it would have been Fred Claire and Kevin Towers."

Barry Axelrod, a sports agent who was one of Towers' closest friends, was also intrigued by the relationship: "I thought, 'Man, how did these two become fast friends?' Fred is so reserved and proper and Kevin is . . . well, in 2009, when he was let go from the Padres by [team executive] Jeff Moorad, one of the things he said about Kevin was that he was too much of a gunslinger—impetuous and impulsive—shooting from the hip and saying whatever came to mind. Kevin didn't take that as an insult. He was a gunslinger, and Kevin went so far as to make that part of his email address. That was Kevin. Fred was more of a button-down, very proper guy."

But appearances also deceived. For starters, the two men shared a deep mutual respect for one another.

"Kevin knew what he didn't know, and he was always trying to learn," Towers' wife, Kelley, said in 2019. "He always had so much respect for people like [UCLA basketball coaching legend] John Wooden, so much respect for people he called the 'sages.' He held Fred in such high esteem. He definitely thought of Fred as a sage."

As general managers, Claire and Towers shared remarkably similar philosophies when it came to roster building, both placing a high premium on team chemistry and looking for players with good work ethics and character.

"The analytics side of baseball that has become so prevalent is based on primarily numbers and on-field performance," Axelrod said. "Frankly, you can have some bad apples who perform very well on the field but who are terrible in a clubhouse. If he was looking to acquire someone, one of the very first questions Kevin asked was, 'What kind of guy is he?' He would spend time looking into that by talking to managers, general managers, agents, media people, clubhouse attendants who are around players day in, day out."

Claire employed an almost identical approach. Both also relied upon and valued contributions from each member of their organizations, from top to bottom.

"Kevin was always about a total team effort," Claire recalled. "I've always felt that if you really want to judge a general manager, ask the people he deals with directly, the scouts, the manager, the minor league managers, the minor league personnel, the major league staff, the players. Ask members of opposing teams. Everyone thought the world of Kevin. You can create a lot of headlines and win championships. Kevin had that success, too. But you can't just judge by those results. Kevin was always about the team and everyone respected him."

Finally, and perhaps most importantly, both Claire and Towers were committed to treating other people with kindness and respect, no matter who they were.

"With Kevin, there was no top of the food chain or bottom of the food chain," Kelley Towers said. "Everyone was the same. He treated the ushers the same way he treated other general managers. It was about helping other people. The hearts of Kevin and Fred were the same. It's just that their approaches to life were different."

In 1998, the year Claire was fired by the Dodgers, Towers' Padres team won the National League pennant, the pinnacle of his career as a front office executive. Towers was the San Diego general manager until he was fired in 2009, and general manager of the Arizona Diamondbacks for four years beginning in 2010. That year, Kirk Gibson was the Diamondbacks' interim manager.

"We just kind of hit it off immediately, and he hired me [as full-time manager]," Gibson remembered in 2019. "I think you could call him an old-school baseball guy who made decisions by the eye. He knew what kind of player he wanted, and he had a nickname for every player. He was unique in that he could say stuff to players like nobody could. He was honest. You knew where he was coming from. And he was very successful.

"And he just loved to spar. You just didn't give him an idea, you had to justify your idea and he was going to challenge you. That was fun. We really had a good time doing that. I remember that we won my first spring training game as the manager and Kevin came in my office. He loved that we won. He loved to wear the horns. That's what he called it, 'wearing the horns.' But when he started talking about the game, he said, 'Dammit. How many times did our pitchers throw over to first base? That was excessive.' I smiled and said, 'You ain't seen nothing yet.'"

Towers, Gibson, and their wives became close friends during their Diamondback years, which ended in 2014. Two years later, the two couples rented a house in the California desert for the Coachella Music Festival.

"We were going to six concerts in three days: Dylan, the Stones, The Who, Neil Young, Paul McCartney, and Roger Waters from Pink Floyd," Gibson remembered. "We had gone through five shows and were exhausted from the music. But we knew that KT wouldn't skip the last show. 'We're here, we're going.' That's how he was. So, we came up with a scheme to convince him to blow off Roger Waters."

Gibson also remembered how frequently that weekend Towers attempted to clear his throat. A short time later, late in 2016, Towers was diagnosed with anaplastic thyroid cancer, a rare form of the disease and one of the most deadly.

"About two or three weeks later he called me and said he had some bad news," Gibson remembered. "He hung on for as long as he could. He was a gamer. He was tough. Even in the toughest of times, he didn't want anybody feeling sorry for him."

•◆•

Though Claire was formally out of the game since 1998, he and Towers had remained in touch over the years. Late in his tenure with the Padres, when San Diego was in town to play the Dodgers, the two began meeting for breakfast at Pie 'n Burger, talking for hours about player evaluation, scouting, clubhouse chemistry, roster construction, and changes in the game.

"When Kevin and Fred got together for breakfast, I never knew how long Kevin would be gone," Kelley Towers said.

Sometimes Bruce Bochy, the Padres manager and Towers' close friend, would join them. At other times, as Claire and Towers conversed at a table in back, Towers' players filled the Pie 'n Burger lunch counter.

It went on that way for several years: two very different personalities but like-minded baseball guys coming together to share their passion for the game. Baseball was the sole basis of their bond until 2016, when the world changed for them both.

•◆•

Fred Claire recognized it the first time he set foot on the City of Hope campus: the understanding between fellow cancer sufferers, a unique empathy often conveyed in very quiet, subtle ways.

"Maybe with just a smile," he said. "One patient with a hospital ID bracelet nodding to another. Maybe a look of caring and compassion. It is an instinct. It is from the heart and unscripted. It is the feeling of being together in the battle against a common opponent, often understood without words being spoken. With cancer comes a knowing that only we as patients can comprehend."

It was true. No one else could fully understand the fear, the exhaustion, the mental and physical pain, the anxiety of looming test results, the moments of great hope and great despair. Even Sheryl Claire, who had been by her husband's side for every moment of his cancer journey, conceded that she couldn't fully appreciate what Fred was going through, at least not like another patient.

"I was there as a caregiver, but I'm not the person who has been in a radiation chamber thirty-three times and suffered the burning from the procedure," she said. "I'm not the one who has had powerful drugs pumped into my veins. As a caregiver, I was always by Fred's side. I could see and all but feel what he was going through. But I wasn't in the chair receiving an infusion or in the hospital bed. Your experience is through your loved one, but I haven't had to face the challenges as a patient. Everyone who has, knows. There is a very strong sense of that."

Kevin Towers knew.

"Of all the friends I have in baseball who reached out to me after my cancer became known, all those people who were so supportive, none of them understood it better than Kevin," Fred said. "There were so many calls from so many people with sincere expressions of concern, but with Kevin it was just that connection. He understood. We understood it together."

As Kelley Towers put it later, "They were teammates in the battle."

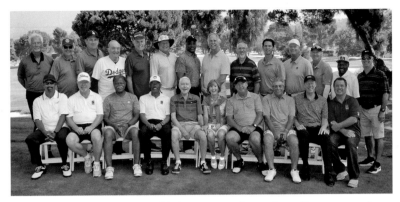

The first Fred Claire Celebrity Golf Classic in 2017 featured an all-star cast and representatives of all five Los Angeles Dodgers teams that have won a World Series title. Proceeds went to City of Hope.

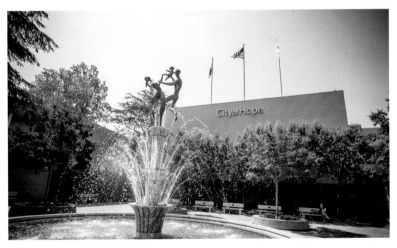

Founded in 1913, City of Hope is a national leader in advancing the research and treatment of cancer.

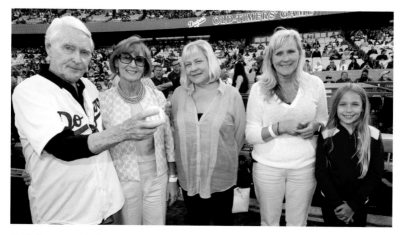

Fred threw out the honorary first pitch in 2017 and was joined by his wife, Sheryl; daughters, Jennifer and Kim; and granddaughter, Tyler.

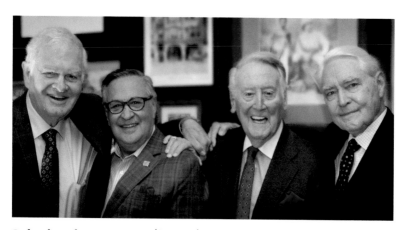

Dodger legendary announcers (from left) Ross Porter, Jaime Jarrin, and Vin Scully provided great support for Fred's golf tournaments to benefit City of Hope.

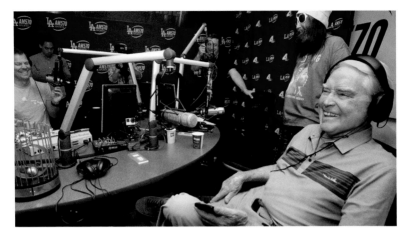

Los Angeles radio station 570 with the team of Petros and Money and Vic "The Brick" Jacobs, who provided great support for Fred's golf events.

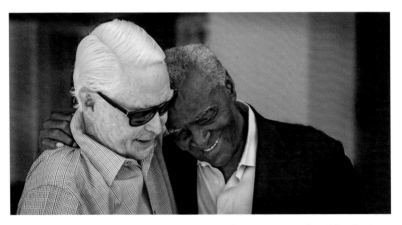

As a great turnout of former Dodgers came together to assist Fred with his fundraising activities, there was a quiet moment with "Sweet Lou" Johnson.

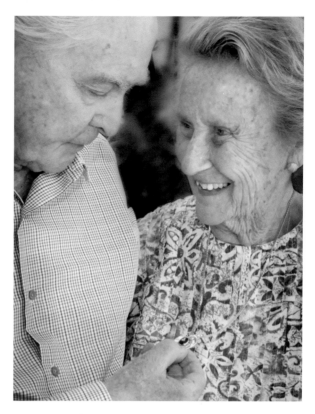

Terry Seidler was in attendance to support Fred and his golf tournaments, and proudly wore a charm from the 1955 World Series, the Dodgers' first ever championship.

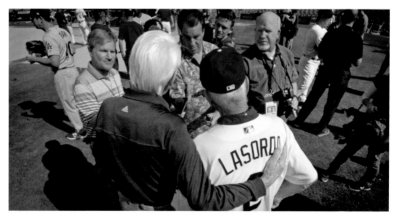

Fred and Tommy Lasorda were back side-by-side when the Dodgers honored Fred at their Oldtimers Game in 2017.

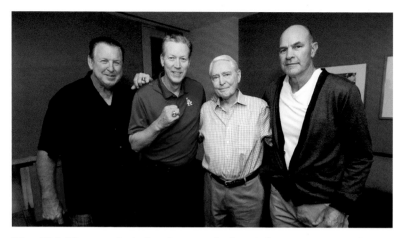

When Kirk Gibson was invited to throw out the first pitch on Opening Day of 2018 at Dodger Stadium, he invited Fred to join him along with Mickey Hatcher and Orel Hershiser.

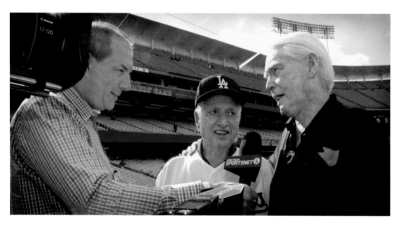

Fred and Tommy reunited in 2017, nearly a half century after they first met at Dodgertown in the Spring of 1969.

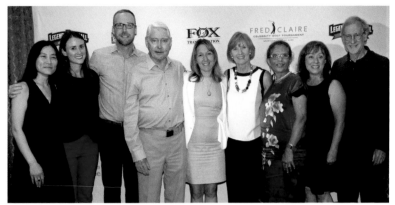

At his first celebrity golf tournament to benefit City of Hope, Fred introduced the medical staff involved in his recovery as, "the greatest team I've ever known."

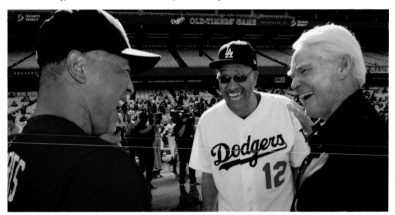

Los Angeles Dodgers manager Dave Roberts and former Dodger great Tommy Davis share a laugh with Fred.

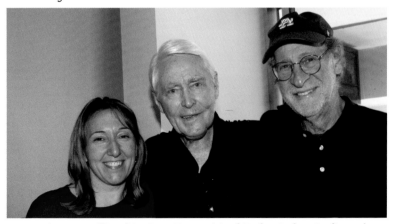

Dr. Eminia Massarelli and Dr. Steve Forman joined Fred at Dodger Stadium when he was honored in a pre-game ceremony in 2017.

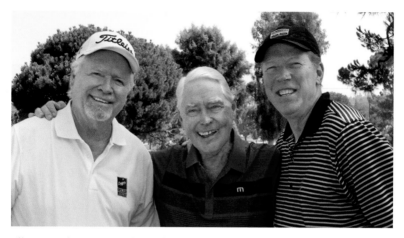

All-time Dodger greats Bill Russell and Orel Hershiser have been supportive of Fred during his recovery from cancer treatment.

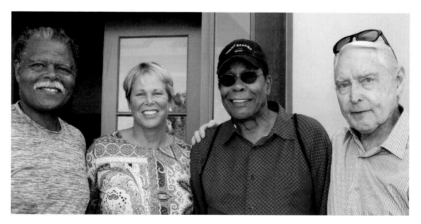

Reggie Smith, Ann Myers Drysdale, and Rod Carew joined Fred for his first celebrity golf tournament. Carew was honored with the first Celebration of Life award.

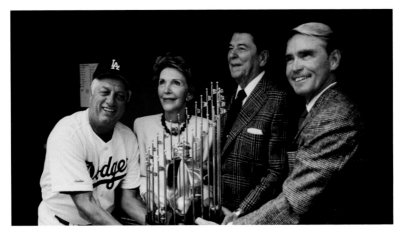

Former President Ronald Reagan and former First Lady Nancy Reagan were at the Dodgers' Opening Day game in 1989 to celebrate the World Championship with Tommy and Fred.

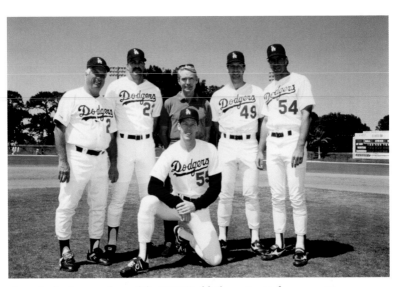

Award-winning members of the 1988 World Champion Dodgers were Tommy Lasorda, Kirk Gibson, Fred, Tim Belcher, Tim Leary, and Orel Hershiser.

• ◆ •

Just a few years before, the return of Fred's squamous cell carcinoma would have been a death sentence. Even with immunotherapy, his survival was a long shot. But even then, Fred said, "I had an understanding that Kevin was fighting a tougher opponent."

When Kevin was diagnosed in late 2016, he was told that his life expectancy was probably measured in months, not years.

"Kevin, being the hard-driving guy that he is, asked, 'How many months? Tell me,'" recalled his friend, Barry Axelrod. "The doctor basically said, 'Well, between two months and two years; probably six months.'"

But Kevin never believed the odds applied to him.

"He confronted it as he did most things, with a competitive spirit," Kelley said. "He was going to beat it. There was no doubt in his mind, and no doubt in my mind, that this was going to be a lesson that we would learn and grow from but ultimately move past."

One day in 2017, not long after he had spoken with Kevin, Kirk Gibson called Fred.

"You and KT are the two toughest sons-of-bitches I know," Gibson said.

"I'll take that as a compliment, coming from you," Fred replied.

By then, Gibson was suffering from Parkinson's disease.

"Oh yeah. They were the toughest," he said in 2019 about Claire and Towers. "They didn't give in. They took great pride in that. That's the way I was, too. We took great pride in it. We would do what we had to do to suck it up."

Kevin and Fred first discussed their shared battle in a phone call on January 18, 2017. Over the next year, in a series of phone conversations and text messages, the two celebrated positive medical reports and comforted each other when the news wasn't good and the suffering was the greatest.

"I was so pleased to hear that things are going better for you," Fred told Kevin in a text in February that year. "Call when you get a chance, and we will catch up."

It was just a few days later that Dr. Gernon discovered new lumps in Fred's neck.

"Between the two of us, [the] doctor found a spot in my neck that likely will require another surgery but [I] remain hopeful," Fred wrote.

Kevin was struggling, too, but told Fred he was hanging in there after being hospitalized for twelve days. "Still battling and don't plan on giving up," he wrote.

On March 25, Fred told Kevin he had received his first immunotherapy treatment the day before: "If the drug or drugs are as good as my immune system has been to me, I will be pleased. We need to believe in our powers of healing and gain inspiration from faith, family, and friends. You are in my thoughts and prayers."

Six days later, Kevin replied, "Taking one day at a time and doing my best to find joy in each day. You are in my thoughts and prayers."

On April 10, Kevin shared a photograph of himself and Bruce Bochy, then the manager of the San Francisco Giants, that had been taken during a recent visit to the San Diego ballpark. Kevin also expressed delight at Bill Plaschke's column about Fred that had been published a few days before: "Nice to see good guys and true professionals get a little credit they deserve. God bless you, Fred. I hope your new treatment is benefitting you."

"One more immunology session and then we wait a short while for a scan," Fred wrote in reply. "Pain is my companion, and I want to shake it. Best part of my day is walking about two miles. Kirk [Gibson] called yesterday and said he has trip to LA coming and may try to stop by with Orel. Good to see you at the park, and I'm going to try to get out more. Need to fight the fatigue along with the pain. You are in my thoughts and prayers."

In mid-May, Kevin wrote to tell Fred he had recently spent several days in the hospital.

On June 2, Fred reported that his cancer had stabilized, apparently in response to his immunotherapy.

Kevin also had good news: "Making some progress with my experimental crud as well, Fred. A few of my tumors that were in my muscle mass have shrunk in size. That is a positive sign. Have a great weekend, Fred!"

On June 10, Fred contacted Kevin before leaving for Dodger Stadium to throw out the ceremonial first pitch and told him he would be in his thoughts.

"Have a great night at park tonight," KT replied. "Still not ready to travel yet, or I would be there."

Two weeks later, Fred invited Kevin and his wife to the first City of Hope golf tournament.

"Going in tomorrow for bunch of scans," Kevin replied. "Hopefully, still shrinking. Still feeling well, Fred. If health continues to improve, I will see you in August. God bless."

"Wishing and praying for good results," Fred wrote. "I had a scan Monday and results showed things are improving related to tumors. Immunotherapy seems to be working, but drugs are causing colitis, and they have backed me off drugs and giving me steroids. Overall the report today was the most encouraging in our one-year journey. How great it would be to have you with us in August. We are all on a journey to celebrate life and help others."

A July 27 message from Kevin brought the best news yet: "Got positive news back today from oncologist who reviewed my scans yesterday. No cancer in bones and many tumors in my body have begun to shrink. Really good news that I wanted to share with you."

"Kevin. There truly are no words to tell you how happy I am with this report," Fred replied. "We are on parallel paths with my good scan on Monday. We are teammates on a winning team with an ultimate goal. And you remain in my thoughts and prayers."

But on August 3, Kevin told Fred that he might not be able to attend the tournament, after all, due to a surgery scheduled on August 8 to remove a small calcified mass blocking the left chamber of his lung. The surgery was a success. "Back home now and breathing much better," Kevin wrote to Fred on August 13. "Don't think I will be able to physically attend your tournament, but I assure you I'll be there in spirit! God bless you and your family."

"You will be with me in spirit tomorrow and forever," Fred replied. "You will have many MLB friends here. YOU ARE RESPECTED DEEPLY because you always have respected the game."

•◆•

By the end of 2017, Fred had turned a corner. His scans were clean and side effects receding. By then, Kevin had far exceeded the life expectation of his doctors and seemed to have battled his disease to a stalemate. Fred wrote Kevin to wish him Happy Thanksgiving on November 23.

"Doing great Fred!" Kevin replied. "Hope you and your loved ones are well."

"Sheryl and I are hoping for the best on a scan result this coming Monday. Life is a treasure, as we know."

Fred's scan was clean. Later during the holidays, Kevin and his wife were able to relax together at a vacation home in the desert, sipping mimosas, hopeful about the year to come. Fred sent his last message to Kevin on January 15. About that same time, Kevin was admitted to a San Diego hospital with fluid on his lungs.

"Once again, he was beating that, too—doctors were set to discharge him," Bob Nightengale wrote in *USA Today*. But on January 30, "He never woke up."

Kevin Towers was just fifty-six years old.

Tributes poured in from across the baseball world when the news of his death became known. One came from Chicago Cubs President Theo Epstein, who in 2016 was the architect of the Cubs' first championship team in more than a century. Epstein had worked for Towers out of college and considered him to be one of his most important mentors.

"When the Chicago Cubs won their first World Series in 108 years in 2016, and Epstein had a private party two months later in January, Towers was one of the first people he invited," Nightengale wrote. "The way Epstein figured it, there would be no party without KT. Towers was his mentor, his role model and the man who helped develop him into one of the game's finest executives."

The lessons from Towers, Epstein said, went far beyond baseball: "He taught me so much about life—how to treat people, how to have the right attitude, how to allow yourself to be happy and enjoy life. I'm not wired that way naturally, but he taught me how to do that.

"In this game, so many people are cutthroat, looking out for themselves, or trying to squeeze the bottom line out of every situation. He was the complete opposite, saw the best in everyone, and tried to help everyone. Who wouldn't want to be around somebody like that?"

In Pasadena, Fred Claire was stricken by the news.

"Just sadness. Just grief. An empty feeling just a terrible, terrible loss," Claire recalled two years later. "There was a very deep relationship, and one that was so personal, that there are just no words to express the loss. I feel it even today."

·◆·

Fred Claire and Kelley Towers had never met until that Sunday afternoon a few weeks after Kevin's death, when the baseball world gathered at San Diego's Petco Park to celebrate the life and spirit of the man known as KT.

Claire introduced himself to Kelley afterward.

"I talked to a lot of people that day, and I was in kind of a fog," she remembered. "But seeing Fred was just such a heart spark, knowing what he had gone through himself. And for him to be there was such an homage to Kevin."

By then, Fred was well into the planning of his second City of Hope golf tournament. He told Kelley that half of the proceeds would be designated for research to find a cure for anaplastic thyroid cancer in Kevin's memory. Fred invited her to attend.

"I don't play golf, but I will be there," Kelley Towers said.

On another radiant Southern California day, August 20, 2018, Kelley Towers' cell phone rang as she started her drive from her home in San Diego to Oakmont Country Club. It was Theo Epstein, unexpectedly checking in. When he learned where she was headed, Epstein donated a day at Wrigley Field to be auctioned off at Fred's tournament.

"Any day I get to carry the flag of Kevin is a good day for me," Kelley remembered. "That day I felt like I was exactly where I was supposed to be."

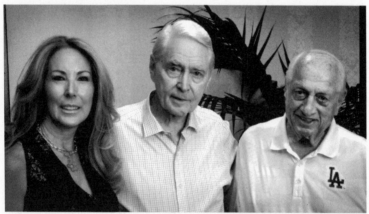

Kelley Towers, widow of former baseball executive Kevin Towers, attended Fred's golf tournament dinner in 2018 when Tommy Lasorda received the Celebration of Life Award.

Fred Claire and Kelley Towers were seated next to each other at the tournament banquet, during which Claire and Dr. Forman presented Tommy Lasorda with the second Celebration of Life Award. During a quiet moment, Fred leaned toward Kelley.

"Kevin is here," he said.

"I know," Kelley replied.

A few weeks later, Dr. Massarelli invited the Claires to the City of Hope Biomedical Research Center, saying there was someone the oncologist wanted them to meet. When they arrived, Massarelli introduced Fred and Sheryl to a young researcher, Atish Mohanty, who had been hired with the proceeds of their benefit golf tournaments. Working under Massarelli, Mohanty was devoted to finding a cure for head and neck and anaplastic thyroid cancer, the disease that had taken Kevin Towers' life.

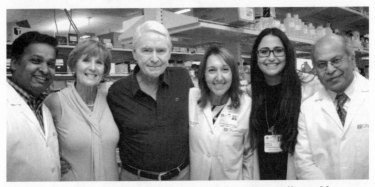

Fund raising efforts by Fred and Sheryl enabled Dr. Massarelli to add a young researcher, Atish Mohanty (left), to the COH team. To Dr. Massarelli's left are research assistant Rebecca Pharaon and Dr. Prakash Kulkarni of the COH Biomedical Research Center.

That day at the research center, Fred and Sheryl listened as Dr. Massarelli described the challenges presented by such a deadly disease with no known cure. That was what made the financial support of people like the Claires so crucial, the oncologist said. As they left the research center that day, the couple each realized—without having to say so—that the day was one of the most meaningful and gratifying of their lives.

10

A VERY GOOD YEAR

O
n October 24, 1988, thousands of euphoric baseball fans lined the streets of downtown Los Angeles to celebrate the Dodgers' World Series championship that had been captured four days earlier. In the boisterous parade, team owner Peter O'Malley rode in the first open-top car with manager Tommy Lasorda and Mayor Tom Bradley. Fred and Sheryl Claire shared the second with postseason hero Mickey Hatcher and his family. Orel Hershiser raised the World Series trophy from his car. He and Kirk Gibson inspired the loudest cheers.

The celebration ended with a City Hall rally. Lasorda summoned Gibson to the podium to once more invoke the team's mantra.

"The fruits of victory!" Gibson bellowed, pumping his fist in the air. "How sweet it is!"

Fred Claire also addressed the happy throng: "The Dodgers were a team with a dream, and we made dreams come true. In

1989, our challenge is clearly before us. Few teams in history have repeated as champions, and our goal in 1989 is to repeat and be there again."

The next year, the Dodgers fell to fourth place instead. Claire had looked forward to other celebrations after future championships, but they were not to be. Yet, thirty years after his first parade, Claire was invited to be part of another—one that might have held even greater significance.

On January 1, 2018, he rose long before dawn and was driven to a staging area of the 129th Rose Parade in Pasadena. The world's finest marching bands were assembling there, along with hundreds of horses from the parade's equestrian units and scores of floats featuring iconic floral arrays.

For the forty-sixth consecutive year, a City of Hope float would be one of the entries. It was titled, "Transforming Lives With Hope" and featured thousands of pink, yellow, and red roses carefully arranged around the float's base. A lush canopy of flowers spilled down.

As parade preparations continued, Fred waited that morning in the predawn chill with Dr. Forman; Fred's surgeon, Dr. Gernon; and Lupe Santana, the patient navigator and, by then, close family friend. Each of them, like Fred, wore matching blue parkas bearing the motto, "The Miracle of Science With Soul." The one City of Hope parade participant who did not was a young major league infielder named Enrique "Kike" Hernandez, who stood out in his white Dodger jersey. Hernandez' connection to City of Hope came through his father, who had been successfully treated for multiple myeloma after consulting with Forman, who put together a treatment protocol (that he largely underwent in Puerto Rico).

But on that Rose Parade morning, the focus was on Claire and ten others who shared the City of Hope float with him—each of them survivors in their respective fights against cancer or diabetes, and people committed to using their experiences to help others.

In another blue parka was Cory Norton, a firefighter suffering from a rare form of spinal cancer. Norton chose to focus not on his misfortune, but on the small army of people who had joined him in his fight.

"It's easy to forget how great people are in this ugly world," Norton said. "I had so many people who I have never met before donate to me, and they were willing to help in any way possible. It really opened my eyes again to see the good."

Rosemary Estrada had prevailed against colon and thyroid cancer at City of Hope and then became involved in efforts to promote cancer awareness. Nicole Allen, a single mother with a long family history of cancer, found her way to City of Hope after another doctor dismissed her health concerns. While being treated at City of Hope for breast cancer, she became a patient advocate, urging others to get second medical opinions. Real estate agent Gary Lorenzini raised money for prostate cancer research after being successfully treated for that disease.

"I had read their biographies and was fully aware that I was just one of eleven, many of them with stories much more dramatic than mine, survivors who had been through much more than I," Fred remembered.

As the sun rose over the mountains, he finally took his place on the float, seated between a young man named Chad Bible, and a thirty-one-year-old woman, Jackie Solano. Bible was a star outfielder at San Diego State University when diagnosed with Hodgkin's lymphoma in January 2017. By that winter morning, he was in remission. Solano had run a half-marathon while being treated at City of Hope for breast cancer.

"Chad and I talked about baseball," Fred recalled. "Jackie and I were both runners, so we had that connection. And we were cancer survivors. Here I was, seated beside two very young people. Wherever my own cancer journey was going to take me, I realized how fortunate and blessed I had been. Cancer did not hit me at eighteen or nineteen or thirty. I was never more appreciative of my life, and I was so inspired by the strength of those two sitting beside me."

Finally, after hours of waiting, the float began to move. The parade had finally begun.

"Then there was the joy of that experience for all of us," Fred remembered. "I knew this was a once-in-a-lifetime opportunity. And who knows how many people watching had a connection to City of Hope? It was very special."

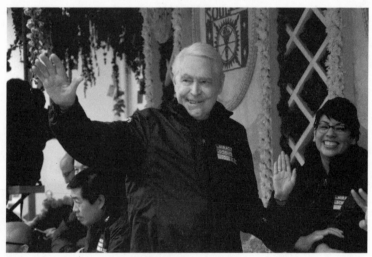

Ten other cancer survivors joined Fred on the 2018 City of Hope float in the Rose Parade. Waving to Fred's left is fellow patient Jackie Solano. The theme of the float was, "Transforming Lives With Hope."

A few miles away, at their home in Pasadena, Sheryl was among the millions who watched the parade on television. She saw her beaming husband who, less than a year before, had been given what amounted to a death sentence. Now there he was in his blue parka, wearing sunglasses on the bright morning, waving at the hundreds of thousands of people who lined the parade route along Pasadena's Colorado Boulevard.

"I had certainly seen Fred on television plenty of times before," she said. "It seemed like he was on TV too much during the Dodger days. But this was different. I was thrilled."

For the Claires, it was a fitting beginning for what would be a very good year.

•◆•

On the evening of February 10, Fred reconnected with Mt. San Antonio College for the first time in nearly a half-century. Mt. SAC, as it is known, is a two-year junior college in the town of Walnut, a community in eastern Los Angeles County. At that night's banquet, Claire was inducted into the school's Athletic Hall of Fame.

To others, the recognition might have seemed a relative footnote to Fred's long life of achievement and accolades. But not to him. He had been born and grown up in a working-class family in a small town in Ohio with a boyhood dream of a life in sports, but without the athletic talent to earn a scholarship or the financial means to attend a four-year university. His path would by necessity start modestly.

"I realized I wanted to be connected with sports," Fred recalled. "That was a driving force in my life, but I could see my athletic talent wasn't going to carry me very far. My interest in writing came about because of my interest in sports. That's how I felt I could stay connected."

Fred's family eventually relocated to Southern California, where he finished high school. In 1954, after a year at El Camino College in the South Bay area of the Los Angeles metro area, Fred enrolled at Mt. SAC when his family moved to the nearby community of Pomona.

"I worked at a small newspaper during the summer after my first year of junior college to pay my tuition," Fred remembered. "I took advantage of my opportunity at Mt. SAC, made good enough grades to get into San Jose State, which had a wonderful journalism program. Eventually I realized I had been very fortunate, and I realized how much that opportunity to go to college meant to me."

On the night of his Hall of Fame induction, a tribute video highlighted the public successes of Fred Claire's Dodger years. But a series of testimonials also emphasized aspects of his life that took place out of the spotlight.

"There is the general way of doing things, and the Fred Claire way of doing things," said Bill Shumard, who was hired by Fred during his Dodger years and went on to become CEO of the Special Olympics of Southern California. "Fred demands excellence, and he demands it from himself first and foremost. I have managed to do pretty well because of Fred's influence on my life."

Sam Fernandez was a young lawyer who joined the Dodgers during Claire's years and later became the Dodger's Executive Vice-President and general counsel. During Claire's time as general manager, the two men sat side by side during player negotiations with agents and while working out contracts.

When Fernandez was honored in 2013 as the Los Angeles County Bar Association's Corporate Counsel of the Year, he asked Fred to present the award in a dinner emceed by Dodger announcer Vin Scully.

"Fred is a gentleman. He's a person of high integrity and totally focused on doing the best job possible," Fernandez said in the video. "Watching the way that Fred conducts himself is an example for all of us."

Fred hired Mike Fox for the Dodger ticket department. Fox went on to run one of Southern California's most successful trucking companies.

"In the ten years that I worked for him, I never saw him in a situation where he fabricated something," Fox said. "It was always transparency. He demanded that. We all learned so much from his leadership. Just have integrity. Have character. Be honest. Do the best you can."

The final tribute came from Jeff Fellenzer, the intern running the Dodger Stadium message board on the day Rick Monday saved the American flag. Fellenzer went on to a successful career in journalism, sports management, and, later, in academia. A year after Fred Claire's career with the Dodgers ended, Fellenzer reached out to his former boss, asking him to be his co-professor at the University of Southern California, teaching a new class on sports and business.

"Fred was a passionate lecturer who spoke from the heart and illustrated his points with compelling, real-life examples from his own long experience as a sportswriter and with the Dodgers," Fellenzer remembered.

But at USC, and in later teaching stints at Long Beach State and Caltech, Fred Claire was known as much for what he did for students outside the lecture hall. The door of his Pasadena office was always open to any young person who sought his counsel.

"He has helped countless students of mine, even after he and I taught together," Fellenzer said in the Mt. SAC tribute video. "They were my students, and to him they were his students because he was my friend. It's been very apparent to me how much he cares, how much he wants to make a difference. He's always taken the high road in life. He does the right thing."

•◆•

A decade came and went, then twenty years, yet the 1988 championship team still had not been honored at Dodger Stadium.

"Some of us were quietly wondering when they were going to have a reunion," said Tim Belcher, the rookie starting pitcher on the championship team. "I think the current Dodger front office people were tired of hearing that the 1988 team was the last to win a World Series, and they didn't want to bring us around until they won another one themselves. Eventually you get to the thirty-year mark, and they probably said, 'Oh, what the hell.' We can't wait forever, or they'll all be dead and gone."

Hence the emotional lunchtime gathering at Dodger Stadium on May 12, 2018. The retired athletes were in late middle age now, with hair that had grayed and thinned and waistlines that had expanded. Some, like Parkinson's disease sufferer Kirk Gibson, battled serious health issues. But as sixteen members of the 1988 Dodgers met each other in the Stadium Club overlooking the field, coming together as a group for the first time in so long, it was as if they had just popped the cork on the clubhouse champagne.

Immediately, the old stories began to be retold. The good-natured ribbing picked up where it had left off thirty years before.

"It was like we were all back on the bus again," ace reliever Jay Howell said.

"That Dodger team was like a family," center fielder John Shelby said in 2019. "Everybody cared for each other, and even though it was just for one year, it felt like we had an everlasting bond. The day when we finally got together showed how strong that bond was. It felt like we had just won the World Series the night before and were celebrating as a team, as a family."

It was an extended family, one that went beyond just the players. One after another, the players embraced manager Tommy Lasorda, then ninety years old. And they gravitated to the man who had assembled the magical ingredients: Fred Claire. Many of the players had heard of Fred's cancer journey and were delighted to see him looking so well. Fred and Sheryl were just as delighted to see them.

"You looked down on the field from where we were in the Stadium Club," Claire remembered. "The field was at its most beautiful and the players could look into the dugout, the place that had been their home. There was Shelby and Rick Dempsey and John Tudor, a tough guy from the Northeast who came up to me and thanked me for bringing him to the Dodgers. Jay Howell knew I had a City of Hope golf tournament coming up and asked what he could do to help. It was just a wonderful togetherness. We celebrated as a team. Not just the players, but everyone from the clubhouse guys to the top of the front office. We were one. We are one. We will always be one."

Thirty years before, it had not gone unnoticed by the players how Claire was in the clubhouse every day, or around the batting cage, and on every road trip, always available to any player who needed to talk.

Tim Belcher said, "A lot of times today, if a GM sends a popular player down or trades a popular veteran or doesn't make a trade the club thinks he should make, he might avoid the clubhouse for a few days to let things calm down. But Fred would walk right through in his normal routine. 'Hey, here I am.' If they had something to say, don't say it in the media, don't backstab. Let's talk about it. I always appreciated that about him, particularly not coming from a playing background. That showed a lot of courage on his part."

"He's such a soft-spoken guy, and he speaks in such measured tones that you don't really get a sense of just how fierce a competitor and how tough a guy he is until you're around him in a baseball setting like I was," Belcher continued. "He was as tough as any player that I played with. He didn't lace them up, obviously, but just his steadfastness in sticking to what he believes in, believing in people and character and hard work. The makeup of our team showed that."

Claire and others could not help but reflect on the series of events that had led to their appointment with history. Belcher compared the 1988 Dodgers to the 1980 Olympic hockey team that shocked the world by winning the gold medal. He said Claire and Team USA coach Herb Brooks employed similar philosophies when assembling their squads.

"The comparisons between us and the Miracle on Ice team are really on target," Belcher said. "Their coach said, 'I don't want the best player. I want the best guy for us.' Not the guy with the best statistics that any guy picking up the sports page could figure out. Fred accomplished that, too. His one big splash was Gibson, but look at the other news he made."

Signing Mickey Hatcher after his release by the Twins;

giving Rick Dempsey another shot; taking a chance on ace reliever Jay Howell, who was coming back from an injury; acquiring the young pitcher Belcher in a trade with Oakland for shortstop Alfredo Griffin; and relief pitcher Jesse Orosco. All were key components of the championship team.

"More than anything, he liked my Midwest upbringing and my toughness and wanted to take a chance on that," Belcher said. "Fred's an Ohio guy himself."

John Shelby might have been the best example of Claire's philosophy.

•◆•

Two years before he was named general manager, Fred Claire was watching a spring training game between the Dodgers and Baltimore, sitting next to close friend and former Dodger player Lou Johnson, when a young Oriole outfielder came to the plate.

"You know, Fred, this guy is quite a player," Johnson said of Shelby. "I know him because we're both from Louisville. He's a great guy and has a lot of talent."

The conversation stuck. Claire remembered it two years later when he was the Dodgers' new general manager in desperate need of a quality center fielder. He heard that Shelby had just been sent down by the Orioles to their minor league team in Rochester, New York.

"I sent scout Mel Didier to Rochester," Claire recalled. "This is late April. Mel is out at the ballpark early every day and he calls me, 'Fred, this guy has just been sent down to the minors, but he's the first guy on the field every day, and it's freezing cold. He's just working as hard as he possibly can.'"

In other words, Shelby was just the kind of player Claire loved. He quickly worked out a trade with the Orioles. The Dodgers had just arrived in New York for a series against the Mets when Claire called Shelby himself.

"I said, 'We've just made a trade, and you are now a member of the Dodgers, and I want you to report tonight,'" Claire remembered. "He said, 'Oh, Mr. Claire, my wife is pregnant, and it will take me two or three days to get to Albuquerque [the Dodgers' top minor league team].' I said, 'John, you're not going to Albuquerque. You are the starting center fielder of the Los Angeles Dodgers.' There was a silence for what seemed like three minutes. Then he said, 'Mr. Claire, I've waited all my life to hear those words.'"

The next day at Shea Stadium, Shelby was in center field for the visitors. The Mets loaded the bases in the first inning for slugger Kevin McReynolds.

"Sheryl and I are there," Claire recalled. "It's the NBC Game of the Week. I can still see it. McReynolds hits a ball that looks like one of those airplanes taking off over Shea Stadium and Shelby goes back and jumps and catches the ball. Sheryl screams, 'He caught it! He caught it!' I kind of calm her down because I know the television cameras could pan our way, and I don't want them to see Sheryl jumping up and down. And I said, 'Sheryl, he's supposed to catch those balls.'"

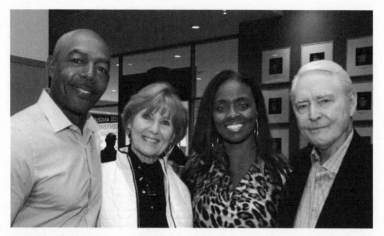

One of Fred's first trades as General Manager in 1987 was to bring John Shelby to the Dodgers from Baltimore. John and his wife, Trina, visited with the Claires during the thirty-year reunion of the Dodgers' World Series Championship in 2018.

For the rest of the season, Shelby was one of the most productive center fielders in baseball. A year later in the National League playoffs, in the epic extra inning game where Orel Hershiser came in with the bases loaded, Shelby would snag another ball off the bat of McReynolds, saving the pivotal Dodger win.

Claire and Shelby embraced when they saw each other on that May afternoon in 2018.

"Any time I hear his name, it brings excitement and joy to me," Shelby said later. "I've probably thanked him a million times for making me a Dodger. He's a class act, a good human being. He treated people fairly. I don't know how you can say anything bad about Fred Claire, and I'm just thankful I had a chance to be a part of what he built. It makes me proud, knowing that I played for him."

• ◆ •

Another Dodger-themed reunion took place three months later at the Oakmont Country Club. Dozens of former players, including Hershiser and Mickey Hatcher, again turned out for the second Fred Claire Celebrity Golf Tournament benefitting City of Hope. Relatives of Jackie Robinson mingled with Jim Campanis, Jr. (Al Campanis' grandson); Kevin Towers' wife, Kelley; and the star-struck eight-year-old son of Dr. Massarelli, Fred's doctor who attended with Drs. Gernon and Forman.

Tommy Lasorda arrived late in the day, dressed in a white golf shirt with the Dodger team logo on the front. Fred Claire was among the first to greet him. Since that magical moment of healing and reconciliation the previous year, on the night Claire threw out the first pitch at Dodger Stadium, his friendship with Lasorda had rekindled and deepened.

The previous September, when the Dodgers celebrated Lasorda's ninetieth birthday at the stadium, Lasorda invited Claire to be one of the speakers. As Claire planned his second benefit golf tournament, Lasorda was his only choice to receive the Celebration of Life Award. In Claire's mind, few others had lived such a life of exuberance and celebration. Few had brought so much happiness to so many.

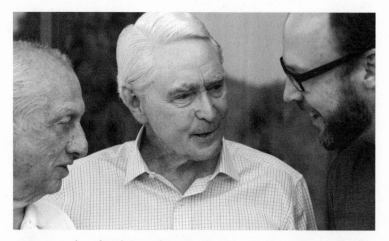

Tommy Lasorda and Fred visit with Dr. Thomas Gernon at the 2018 Fred Claire Celebrity Golf Classic at Oakmont Country Club in Glendale.

At the tournament banquet, Lasorda sat at a table with the Claires, Kelley Towers, and Dodger Vice President Sam Fernandez. From the podium, Fred Claire paid tribute to Kevin Towers, thanked Kelley Towers for attending, and spoke of his old friend.

"Tommy said it best," Fred began. "If you want to achieve a goal, you get everyone on one end of the rope and you pull, and if you pull hard enough, you will achieve your goal, as Tommy did many times. Our goal tonight is to pull down cancer, and we are all at one end of the rope."

After his introduction by Dodger broadcasting legend Ross Porter, applause showered Lasorda as he shuffled to the podium. Speaking haltingly, he thanked Porter and said, "To be here with Fred and a lot of the others, it brought back many, many wonderful times. I'm getting to the point now where I'm getting old. I want to live to be a hundred."

More applause filled the banquet room.

"And with that, the day I get to be a hundred, I'm going to fight the first guy I run into."

Lasorda's audience roared with laughter.

"I'm so happy to see Fred is good and healthy and what the hospital has done for him, which of course he will never forget. And Fred, you put in a lot of hard work to build that championship team. I made them play, but you brought them here."

In the audience, sitting between his wife and Kelley Towers, Fred Claire listened, his eyes brimming with tears. So many things that were sacred to him seemed to come together as Lasorda spoke—their long friendship . . . the joyous memories of 1988 . . . his love for Sheryl and his family . . . his friendship with Kevin Towers . . . his miracle at City of Hope.

At the podium, Lasorda found Hatcher, who was sitting a few feet away.

"Mickey and the rest of you, I don't know how many of you are here, but standing here gives me the opportunity to say, 'Thank you,'" Lasorda said. "You know, a manager needs players who give their heart and soul for the game, and Mickey and so many of the other guys sitting out there tonight, you should be proud of what you have accomplished. I want to say God bless you and take care of yourselves. And to all of you people, continue helping the hospital because it is great. Thank you, Fred."

The crowd stood as the legendary Dodger manager smiled and waved.

•—•

On October 9, 2018, top administrators, doctors, and researchers gathered in a crowded auditorium on the City of Hope campus. Fred and Sheryl Claire were there, too. At the medical center's annual leadership conference, Fred was the featured speaker.

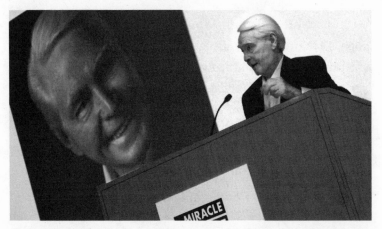

Fred was the speaker at the City of Hope Leadership Conference in 2019. "The one constant theme I've seen . . . at City of Hope is seeing firsthand the people who truly care about patients," said Claire.

In his speech, he noted that, just the week before, James Allison had shared the Nobel Prize for his work in immuno-therapy research. Without it, Fred said, he would not be alive.

"It was the recommendation and then the treatment of immunotherapy that enables me to be here today," he said. "It was really the only option. It was a life-saving option."

But as much as the scientific advances, it was the City of Hope that Fred chose to emphasize that day.

"The one constant theme I have seen play out during our experience at City of Hope is seeing firsthand the people who truly care about patients," he said. "The wording resonates with me because of what a great pitching coach told me one day when I asked how he was able to assist pitchers who were struggling. 'Fred,' he said, 'you have to show them that you care before you tell them what you know.'

"In Major League Baseball, games are sometimes referred to as crucial or even matters of life and death," Claire continued.

"No, it's not life and death. What you do in your roles at City of Hope is a matter of life and death. I refer not just to the doctors and nurses and those involved in radiology and research. It is the volunteers. It is the people who help the patients check in when entering City of Hope. It is the staff that draws blood samples. It is the people working in the records department. It is the people who are involved in the business operations, in fundraising, in event planning, in the pharmacy, in social media, marketing and publicity, and, yes, even the people in the cafeteria and at Starbucks."

He concluded by speaking of the wisdom that only great suffering can bring.

"What I have gained in the last two years at City of Hope goes far beyond anything I thought possible," he said. "I have gained a true appreciation for the blessings of life. The love I have felt from my wife, Sheryl; my children, Jeff, Jennifer, and Kim; and friends has lifted me to the highest level of my life. The spiritual faith I have found in the darkest of days will never dim, and the opportunity to support City of Hope is my greatest achievement. I have been blessed with a competitive spirit, and it is the support from family and friends that drives me to know I am not a victim. I will never be a victim."

That conviction would again be put to the test a few months later, in March 2019, when Fred Claire's agony returned.

11

STRAIGHT OUT OF HOLLYWOOD

In the spring of 2018, a man named Tom Quinley was battling both terminal lung cancer and deepening despair.
The disease had deprived him of his lifelong love—coaching high school baseball—and stolen most of his energy. As he
trudged into City of Hope that day, accompanied by his close
friend, John Sherrard, Quinley wore a green South Hills High
School ballcap. He was attached to a portable oxygen tank
through a breathing tube.

"He just didn't like his life," Sherrard recalled in 2019. "He
knew the quality of life wasn't there. He was tired of that life
and what he was going through."

But his suffering lifted that day, if only temporarily. Quinley
and Sherrard had just stepped into the elevator for a ride to
the second-floor offices of his oncologist, Dr. Massarelli, when

an older, white-haired man and his wife joined them. The man immediately asked about Quinley's cap.

"What does the SH stand for?"

Quinley said he was a baseball coach at South Hills High School in West Covina, a community in the foothills of the San Gabriel Mountains. The man's face brightened with recognition. He said he was familiar with South Hills baseball, the high school powerhouse that had produced major leaguers like Jason and Jeremy Giambi and Cory Lidle. Then the man on the elevator introduced himself.

"I'm Fred Claire. I worked for the Dodgers for thirty years."

Quinley and Sherrard did a doubletake.

"He didn't have to finish the sentence," Sherrard said. "We knew who Fred Claire was."

The conversation between Claire and Quinley took off from there, continuing as they stepped from the elevator and strolled slowly down a hall toward the office of Massarelli, whom Fred knew well, since she was also his oncologist. In that short time, the two strangers discovered a commonality beyond cancer: the game.

"I don't care if you are a general manager of the Dodgers or a high school baseball coach," Fred said later. "You are a baseball guy. I mean this from the bottom of my heart. There is no difference. Tom spent forty years in the game. He devoted his life to the game. It was an honor for me to speak to him because of what he gave, what he achieved, and how he had influenced the lives of so many young people."

•◆•

He was known as Quinner, a native Iowan and lifelong Yankees fan who wore the number eight on the back of his jersey because it had belonged to his favorite player, Yogi Berra. Over a four-decade career at a handful of Southern California highs schools, Quinley coached ten major leaguers and won multiple championships.

"He was a very good tactician, very smart when it came to the game," said Darren Murphy, the head baseball coach at South Hills and one of Quinley's closest friends. "His teams won games that they shouldn't have won. All the best coaches have their teams playing their best at the end, and his teams were very difficult to beat at the end of the season."

But it wasn't Quinley's record of wins and losses that the legion of his former players remembered most.

"Nobody had relationships with his players like Tom did, from just loving them to helping them out through tough situations," said Murphy, who himself had played for Quinley through Little League and high school. "He took care of young men and made sure their lives weren't changed forever because of a mistake. Numerous kids you talk to, when they get to be twenty-five or thirty years old, come back and say, 'Tom came and got me out of jail one night,' or 'I called Tom because I couldn't drive home.' At the time you played for Tom, he really made you feel like you were his favorite. Then you realize there were numerous other kids who felt the same way."

Quinley was the first to suggest to a teenager named Chris Woodward that the young player's hard work and passion for baseball could someday translate into a career in the major leagues. That was a life-changing endorsement for Woodward, who lacked self-confidence at the time. Quinley also played a pivotal role in Woodward's life in ways that had nothing to do with baseball. Woodward's parents divorced when he was young, and Quinley stepped in to fill a void in the player's life.

"My dad wasn't around a whole lot, and Tom knew that," Woodward remembered. "I didn't understand what was going on, but he did. He would always call me and say, 'Hey, you want to field some ground balls? You want to take some batting practice?' He kept me out of trouble in a lot of ways because he knew how much I loved to practice and how much I loved to play baseball. He was just always there."

Woodward went on to a twelve-year career as a major league infielder. He was the third base coach for the Dodgers for three years and then hired as the manager of the Texas Rangers in 2018.

"When I got the managing job in Texas, one of the first things I asked was, 'Does anybody with the Rangers wear number eight? Nobody had it," said Woodward, who wore that number for years as a tribute to another famous eight: Baltimore Orioles shortstop Cal Ripken. "It was a pretty cool moment. I still idolized Ripken, but now it was about wearing Tom's number. It's about Tom. I take a lot of pride when I see that eight now."

Yet Quinley cringed when former players like Woodward praised him publicly. The intensely private, lifelong bachelor hated the limelight and was happiest when he was alone, watering the infield grass or hitting practice grounders to his players.

"He just didn't like the attention," Woodward said. "It's bizarre. It's not normal for people to not want any kind of notoriety for doing something good. It's just who we are as people, right? We care about number one. Most people, on the selfish-selfless scale, tend to be much more on the selfish side. Tom wasn't a perfect person. Nobody is. But he was the most selfless person I've ever known. I can honestly say that."

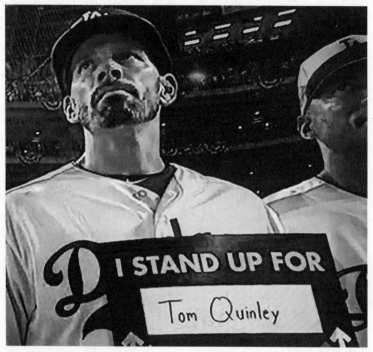

Chris Woodward, now the manager of the Texas Rangers, held up a plaque bearing the name of his high school coach, Tom Quinley, during a StandUpToCancer ceremony at the 2018 All-Star Game, when Chris was a member of the Dodgers' coaching staff.

Quinley died on August 25, 2018, at the age of sixty-four. Woodward and Murphy were among the small group of friends who were with him in the final days.

"Tom was a tough old guy, very proud, but with this disease it was very interesting to see him be vulnerable with a select few," said Murphy. In 2013, when Quinley left his last head-coaching job, Murphy hired him as his South Hills assistant. "He would love you and take care of you and be there for you in the toughest times, but he was never vulnerable himself until he got into the later stages. It was really hard to see, but it was very nice to hear him say things that you wouldn't have expected him to say. He gave a few of us letters at the end. He did tell us that he loved us. That wasn't something you heard Tom say. And you know, as he was getting more and more sick, I'm very happy—and I'm sure others are—that we got to say how we felt."

Woodward, then the third base coach for the Dodgers, saw Quinley a few days before his death.

"He was sleeping most of the time," Woodward recalled. "You didn't really get any reaction from him. Several of us were standing around talking about the Dodgers, who were struggling at the time. I mentioned something about the way we were playing, and Tom kind of perks up. He said, 'Chris, come over here.' We're thinking, 'Oh, Tom's awake.' Then he said something about the team. 'Are you guys [the Dodgers] going to be okay?' I said, 'Yeah. We're going to be okay. The guys are fighting.' He said, 'All right.' Now Tom, he obviously did swear quite a bit, and he comes out with this statement: 'The effing Dodgers are killing me.' I mean, he was on his deathbed. We all just died laughing. It was just perfect Tom. Truth at the very end. This guy is in his last few days on Earth, and that's what he was thinking about. It was a beautiful moment for all of us because it was perfect for all of us to hear that and see that."

• ◆ •

A few months earlier there had been a second and final conversation between Quinley and Fred Claire, this one in Massarelli's waiting room at City of Hope. Fred was thriving after the miracle of immunotherapy, but Quinley was confined to a wheelchair. But that was beside the point during an animated, hour-long conversation about baseball. John Sherrard, the public address announcer and statistician for South Hills baseball, had again accompanied Quinley to City of Hope. He and Sheryl Claire were content to sit and listen.

"It was a conversation that I will never forget," Sherrard recalled. "Tom was a baseball historian, and it was huge because of what Fred means to the sport of baseball. Here is Fred and Tom, two baseball people and career people from different levels, just talking baseball, talking Dodgers. I'm sure the Yankees came up and South Hills. A lot of subjects were covered."

The conversation ended when Quinley was called in for his appointment. The two shook hands and exchanged contact information. Quinley and Sherrard talked about Fred on the way back to their car that day and for the duration of the ride home. Once again, the game had helped lift the weight of Quinley's despair. There was something sacred about two suffering men coming together by chance to jointly celebrate one of the great blessings of their lives.

"You see two people going through what they went through and the connection of baseball," Sherrard recalled. "This is something that is huge. They could forget what they were going through for that one hour. It's very emotional for me because they both had bad situations, and in a few minutes, they would be walking into a doctor's office. One of them might live, and the other was not going to. But here they were talking baseball. That's what baseball does to people in life. Cancer was never mentioned. There was no need."

• ◆ •

Baseball had been at the heart of Jaylon Fong's life since he was old enough to tag along to Little League games with his older brother, Aaron. With his passion for the game, the younger boy quickly became a standout player himself. One day, just before Thanksgiving in 2008, eight-year-old Jaylon had been out playing ball with friends when he returned to the family home in West Covina, complaining uncharacteristically of a headache. He also had a fever and nagging pain in his hip.

His pediatrician, Dr. Leila Jabaji, told Jaylon's parents that the pain and fever were probably the result of a common childhood infection that would run its course in a few days. But the fever lingered for two weeks.

"She said, 'That's not normal. Let me do some blood tests to see if there is anything else there,'" Jaylon's father, Francis Fong, remembered. "She does the blood test in the morning and later that evening I get a call from her on my cell phone. I'm like, 'Why is she calling at this hour?' She said, 'Is Jaylon okay?' I said, 'Yeah, he's fine.' She said, 'We got the blood results back and his platelet counts are abnormal.' I had no idea what she was talking about."

The doctor asked the father to bring Jaylon back to her office the following day to repeat the blood tests. Jabaji had tears in her eyes when she delivered the latest results.

"Imagine your pediatrician telling you with tears in her eyes that something is wrong," Francis Fong remembered. "She said that she had sent Jaylon's blood results to an oncologist. I said, 'Whoa. Why are you sending Jaylon's results to an oncologist?' She said, 'This just doesn't look right.' She kept apologizing. She said, 'I wish I was wrong, but this is not right. He has a big problem, and you have to go to City of Hope right away.'"

A pediatric oncologist, Dr. Lisa Mueller, delivered the devastating news in her City of Hope office a day later. Jaylon had a disease called acute lymphoblastic leukemia.

"It was me, my wife, Melinda, and Grandma in the room with Jaylon," Francis Fong recalled. "At that point there was crying everywhere. Jaylon wasn't sure what was going on. He was just sitting there. But in the same breath, the doctor said he was going to be fine, that he had the most curable type of childhood leukemia. She said, 'I've treated patients who have gone off to college. I have patients now who have their own families and their own kids. We're going to get through this. It's just going to be life-changing for the next three-and-a-half years.' I really appreciated the way she told us. I didn't really hear it at the time. I didn't process it until later on, but she was telling us that he was going to be fine."

The three-and-a-half years of chemotherapy at City of Hope were fairly tolerable for Jaylon, who managed to avoid long hospital stays and miss only a few days of school. He was able to regain enough strength that he could occasionally return to the baseball field. In fact, shortly after he had completed his treatment, he was in the middle of a Little League tournament when Jaylon and his family received more devastating news. Tests showed the chemotherapy had failed to eradicate all of the cancer cells. The boy would have to undergo another two years of treatment.

"For us as parents, it was a punch in the gut," Francis Fong remembered. "It was like getting to the mountain top and getting kicked off. We felt that Jaylon went through everything with flying colors. If this was a test, he would have gotten straight

As through the whole three-and-a-half-year process. Then you hear, 'Sorry, you have to do it all over again.'"

The only person who did not seem devastated was Jaylon himself, now eleven years old and a left-handed pitcher.

Francis Fong said, "So, we were sitting in his doctor's office, and one of his doctors told us that it was a relapse. Jay is sitting there on the table. We told him, 'Jaylon, you're going to have to go through this all over again.' He looked at us and the doctor and said, 'Okay. I have baseball practice at eight tonight.' That was his attitude. He sat out the next couple of games that weekend but came back for the championship game. It was like a movie script. Bases loaded, bottom of the last inning. He comes in to close out the game and strikes out the last batter. That was incredible. I still think about that."

The next two years of treatment were excruciating for the boy and his family, much more so than the first round, with both chemotherapy and radiation treatments that required extended hospital stays. Baseball was out of the question.

"That was the hardest thing for me," Jaylon remembered years later.

Fortunately, the second round of treatment eradicated the disease, and the thirteen-year-old slowly was able to return to the baseball diamond, at first just to cheer on his teammates. Most everyone believed that five grueling years had taken away any chance that Jaylon might someday pitch on the varsity team at South Hills High School.

"You could sense that he had the heart to play, but his body would just give out," Francis Fong said. "He was just happy to be in the dugout. There were games where he just sat in the dugout and watched his teammates. For us as parents, that was enough. We didn't expect him to play; we were very satisfied for him to be healthy enough to come back and just stand on the mound. But early on we realized that's not what he wanted. He wanted to do more than that. He wanted to go out there and be better than everybody else. He exceeded our expectations through sheer will."

By his junior year, Jaylon earned a spot as a pitcher on the South Hills junior varsity team. That year, he occasionally crossed paths with Tom Quinley, the varsity assistant coach battling lung cancer at the same medical center where Jaylon had been treated.

"We really didn't talk about it too much," Jaylon recalled later. "It was mainly just a thing where he would ask me how I was doing and I would ask him how he was doing."

That was typical of Quinley, who never brought up his illness around the team.

"He was a proud man," Francis Fong said. "He really didn't want anyone to feel sorry for him, and he really didn't talk too much about his illness to anybody. He didn't want any visitors at City of Hope, but he knew of Jaylon's story. He told me it really inspired him to see a young kid fight through it."

In the late summer of 2018, Jaylon joined his teammates at Tom Quinley's funeral. Darren Murphy, John Sherrard and others associated with the South Hills program, immediately began making plans to honor the beloved coach by retiring Quinley's number before the first varsity game the following season.

The next January, South Hills traveled to Hawaii for a series of preseason games, during which Murphy and his coaches attempted to sort out their pitching staff.

"When we went to Hawaii, we decided that we had to give

Jaylon a legitimate shot," Murphy recalled. "Other pitchers had greater velocity on their fastballs or a sharper break on their curves, but what Jaylon does is that Jaylon competes. That's the big thing with Jaylon."

The young lefthander surprised his coaches in Hawaii.

"He threw really well," Murphy said. "He threw a bunch of strikes, and he kept the team involved behind him. So, we left Hawaii saying Jaylon is going to be one of our top kids."

The season opener against Rialto Carter High School was scheduled for February 6, 2019. Leading up to the opener, South Hills' top starting pitcher remained sidelined by injury.

"I told our pitching coach, and he agreed, that Jaylon is our number one kid now," Murphy remembered. "And so obviously, Opening Day, Jaylon is going to throw. He worked his way into being the one. He earned the right to be in the discussion, and he made it an easy decision with the fact that it was the day we were honoring Tom. He deserved it, but that kind of added a bit of spice to the story.

"And when you go through what he's gone through, pitching on Opening Day is not going to scare that kid."

A few days before the opener, the coach gathered his team in the dugout after practice.

"He told me in front of the whole team," Jaylon remembered. "I was really surprised."

It seemed a story straight out of Hollywood, just an hour's drive away. On the day South Hills retired Tom Quinley's number, the starting pitcher would himself be a two-time cancer survivor, a senior making his first appearance as a varsity player.

•◆•

In an emotional pregame ceremony, when a new flagpole mal-
functioned, players draped a flag bearing Quinley's number over
the outfield fence. A Kenny Chesney ballad called "Coach" played
over the public address system. After the national anthem,
Jaylon Fong took the mound.

In the stands, Francis and Melinda Fong and their three
other children sat near Tom Quinley's two brothers.

"I had butterflies, but they weren't any greater than for any
other game," Francis Fong recalled. "Every time he steps on the
mound, I get very emotional, regardless of the game situation.
It just brings back the memories. It's a reminder of where Jaylon
has come from."

Jaylon masked his own nervousness beneath a typically
stoic demeanor.

"I knew I was pitching on the day that we were honoring
Coach Quinley, and for me, personally, it was big because it was
my first varsity start," Jaylon remembered. "There were a lot
of nerves."

Murphy expected his starting pitcher to last three or four
innings at the most. Then Jaylon started retiring opposing
hitters in rapid succession, coaxing them into weak ground balls
or harmless pop ups.

"He gets through the first inning and the second inning,"
Murphy remembered. "Then you get into the third inning and
you're like, 'He's throwing a gem here.' All of a sudden, we're in
the fourth inning and he's throwing up zeros. We're getting into the
fifth and we're getting into the sixth, and the whispers start on the
bench: 'I can't believe he's doing this on the day we honored Tom.'"

At the end of six shutout innings, Murphy asked Jaylon how he felt.

"I'm tired," the pitcher conceded.

Another South Hills pitcher, Joshua Ward, was brought in to record the last three outs of a 6–0 victory.

"It was Tom's story to start, but when people left, they were talking about Jaylon *and* Tom," Murphy said. "Then it just took on a life of its own."

• ◆ •

The story of Jaylon Fong and Tom Quinley was featured on television sportscasts and in newspapers across Southern California.

Fred Claire was stunned as he sat in his Pasadena home, having just read about what had happened on the South Hills baseball diamond. Until that February morning, he had not known that Tom Quinley had died, much less that South Hills had planned to retire his number. Add in the story of the young cancer survivor's pitching performance on that special day and it was almost too much to believe.

A few days later, Darren Murphy was caught by surprise when listening to his voicemail messages.

"I was eighteen years old in 1988," he said. "Growing up in Southern California, that was my life right there, the 1988 Dodgers, and all of a sudden, the general manager from that time is calling me. He leaves a message. It was pretty exciting knowing that you're going to be talking to someone who has that history in the game."

When Murphy and Claire eventually spoke, the former general manager asked if he could visit South Hills and speak to Jaylon and the team. Murphy sensed that Claire's offer had something to do with what he had been through himself in the last few years.

"I didn't know Fred at all beforehand," Murphy said. "I would have been interested to talk to him before he had cancer. I know he was always known as genuine and a very nice man. But I felt like the things he had been through had made an imprint on his life. The way he was talking, I gathered that he's probably more thankful than ever about life and about the things he gets to do. I felt that on the phone. He's a busy man, but Tom's story and Jaylon's story touches him now, probably touches him differently than it would have before he was diagnosed.

"To reach out and for him to come and spend a day with us at South Hills High School, that was one of the highlights of my career. That was a very special day."

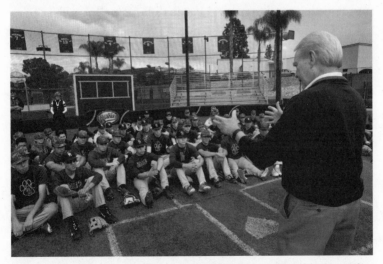

Fred spoke to the South Hills High team in 2019 in honor of Coach Tom Quinley, who lost his life to cancer. "There are two things I want you to think about," Fred said to the team. "I want you to think about what Coach Quinley meant to you and what you can do to help someone else."

It was a hazy March afternoon in the San Gabriel Valley when Fred Claire stepped onto the pristine baseball field of the South Hills Huskies. Dozens of young players sat in a semicircle around home plate in their green caps and green practice jerseys. Darren Murphy was the first to speak.

"How many times do you have a former general manager from the major leagues come out and speak to you, let alone the Los Angeles Dodgers general manager who was the general manager in 1988 when they won the World Series?" Murphy said. "We're still waiting for another one."

The players applauded as Claire came forward to shake Murphy's hand. Claire spoke first about meeting Quinley at City of Hope, how he noticed the green cap on the ailing coach's head, and how Quinley said he coached high school ball at South Hills.

"He didn't say more than that, but he was a baseball man, and I'm a baseball man, and baseball is a small world," Claire said. "So, we struck up an immediate friendship. We met one other time. In talking to the coach, he never talked about his accomplishments. I wouldn't have known if he had ever won a game, let alone a league title, let alone many of them. You know, that's who he was. He only talked about the enjoyment that he had in working with the kids. He didn't say anything about winning. He didn't say anything about his accomplishments. I could see that he loved what he was doing."

The players listened in rapt silence.

"I was very impressed with Coach Tom and very saddened to learn that he had passed away," Claire continued. "Then to see that on Opening Day, that you paid tribute to Coach Quinley and retired his number. I was just really so pleased that you would do that, because he represented so many great things about our game."

<figure>174</figure>

Claire asked the team to offer a few minutes of silence.

"There are two things I want you to think about," Claire said. "I want you to think about what he meant to you, and most importantly, remembering him, what you can do to help someone else."

The boys bowed their heads. The only sound on the high school baseball diamond was birdsong and the California breeze. Claire finally broke the silence: "I've seen enough players and known enough players that I know what I look for. The most underrated part of a scouting report is character. The great coach, John Wooden, who was a friend, said, 'Reputation is what people think you are; character is what you are when no one is looking.' So, when I come out to a field, I want to see how each of you approach the game. I want to see how you are interacting with your coach, with your teammates, with the umpires. I want to see what you put into the game."

Sheryl Claire had been listening from behind the players. Her husband introduced her as she stepped forward and handed Fred a new baseball.

"She is always by my side," he said, and the boys applauded.

Then Fred read what he had inscribed on the ball.

"To the South Hills High School team, in honor of a true champion, coach Tom Quinley, number eight."

The ball bore the signatures of Fred Claire and Kirk Gibson.

For a few minutes more, Claire took questions and told stories from the championship season and his Dodger days. He shook hands and talked with Jaylon Fong.

"He talked to me mostly about baseball and asked me about my favorite pitchers," Jaylon remembered. "I said, 'Clayton Kershaw and Greg Maddux.' He said, 'Those are good choices.'"

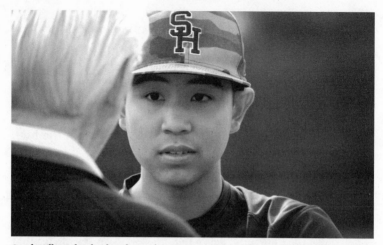

South Hills High School pitcher Jaylon Fong, a two-time cancer survivor, and Fred visited in 2019. The former Dodger executive met with the South Hills team to pay tribute to their late coach, Tom Quinley, whom Fred had met as a fellow patient at City of Hope.

Then Fred and Sheryl Claire disappeared into the hazy afternoon—straight out of Hollywood.

"Tom wasn't around as much the last year, so we had some kids that didn't really know him," Murphy said. "But then the Dodger general manager comes out, and all of a sudden you've got their attention. This guy with a lot of clout starts talking about a good friend of yours and a former coach at the school. Fred helped tell the story of Tom to a lot of the new kids. For them to hear Fred talk about how he and Tom had talked, and how Tom always talked about the kids—that just kind of wrapped it up. It was a good finish to the story."

Before Claire left the field that day, he handed Murphy a stack of business cards.

"He told me to give them to the kids," Murphy said. "If any of the kids needed anything, they could give him a call."

12

HOW WE HANDLE THE CHALLENGES

For most cancer survivors, even after long periods of remission and good health, the fear of recurrence never goes away. Each strange ache, however minor, can inspire a flutter of anxiety; every headache or new bruise becomes a source of concern.

So, Fred Claire could not help but wonder. On Friday, March 15, 2019, after more than a year of steadily improving health, and with reasonable hope that the greatest agonies were behind him, he noticed a puffiness on the left side of his jaw, the area that had been targeted by radiation three years earlier. By Saturday the swelling was unmistakable. Sheryl Claire became concerned on Sunday morning. By that afternoon, when Fred's jaw continued to balloon, she texted Dr. Gernon, who was also concerned and promised to meet the Claires at City of Hope the next morning.

By early evening, what had been numbness in Fred's jaw became excruciating pain. He began to vomit and run a fever. Sheryl's panic grew. Their trip to City of Hope could not wait until morning.

"I was frantic," she recalled. "I was scared. I can remember racing to City of Hope that Sunday and not even getting Fred to the front door without assistance. An attendant helped me get Fred out of the car and into the hospital because she could see I was absolutely panicked."

Fred was admitted to the City of Hope hospital that night and an emergency scan was scheduled for the next day. Doctors soon delivered the good news. There was no sign of cancer. The swelling, pain, and fever were most likely due to an infection.

Sheryl's fear dissolved into relief.

"I have a tendency, when a doctor tells you it is not cancer, to ask to have the words repeated," she said. "It was very reassuring."

Her husband's reaction was more equivocal.

"That's not to say you don't feel relieved when you hear that it's not cancer, but I'm not jumping up and down with joy," Fred remembered. "When your jaw is swollen and you're throwing up and you're running a fever, this is not normal. I think I know my body. I'm not okay. You think you're going good, and now you're not. It might not be cancer, but it was something else that felt pretty serious."

It was. That Sunday was the beginning of a five-day hospital stay. For the Claires, the months to come would be among the most painful and exhausting of their long journey at City of Hope.

"It was really a year on a treadmill that we couldn't seem

to get off," Fred Claire said. "It was almost a replica of 2017. We thought we were off to a great start and we found ourselves in trouble."

•◆•

The email to Fred Claire was written in the early morning hours by another City of Hope patient. Fred's longtime friend, Lisa Bowman, was fighting a relapse of a ferocious form of breast cancer.

"I completed my second round of chemo yesterday," Lisa wrote to Fred that morning in late March 2019. "Those are long days, aren't they? But I was able to flourish under the tender care of my nurse, Annie. We move to Arkansas on Sunday. Chuck [her husband], the dog and I will arrive on April 3. I'm flying back here for the last two rounds. Dr. [Sayeh] Lavasani [a City of Hope oncologist] spent twenty minutes yesterday just looking up oncologists for me, located near our new home. How many physicians do that these days? Extraordinary."

Fred responded with the news of his latest medical setback and reported: "I was released last Friday afternoon, and now I'm on antibiotics as the doctors figure next steps. I'm so pleased to hear of your report and praying for your good health. I'll keep you posted and I feel positive. Best, Fred."

"Oh, Fred. Not what I expected to hear. I will pray," Lisa replied a few hours later. "It is my privilege to journey with you. I'm going to vespers tonight and will place your name before the Lord as part of the group. We're small and tightly connected— and one was a nurse at COH! Be well. I know you are patient. May you find joy in each day. Peace, Lisa."

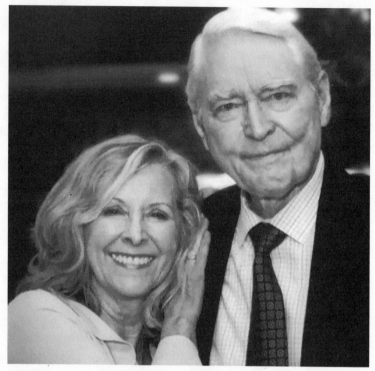

Former radio celebrity Lisa Bowman and Fred reunited at the 2019 awards luncheon of the Southern California SportsBroadcasters Association. Fred encouraged Lisa to get a second opinion at City of Hope.

The two of them had met thirty-six years before in the press box at Dodger Stadium. At the time, Fred was the team vice president in charge of marketing and public relations, which included the media. Lisa was new to the beat as part of the radio coverage for KABC, which provided radio broadcasts of Dodger games.

"I had no sports background," Lisa remembered, "so it was difficult for a few of the experienced sports writers in the press box to accept the neophyte that I was. When Fred walked in, there was just this sense of peace. He was always kind and considerate, so from the first time I met him I kind of knew he was special. He's an unusually gentle man."

The two saw each other only occasionally after Lisa left the Dodger beat and Fred was promoted to general manager. Their fateful reunion occurred on January 28, 2019, at the awards luncheon of the Southern California Sports Broadcasters Association at Lakeside Golf Club. Fred attended with Rich Kee to support close friend Ann Meyers Drysdale, who was being inducted into the organization's Hall of Fame. Claire and Kee pulled into the parking lot of Lakeside at the same time as Meyers Drysdale.

"It was a very warm moment," Fred recalled of their greeting.

A few minutes later, when Fred found his seat at a table in the banquet room, he spotted Lisa walking in his direction with the aid of a cane.

"It wasn't the same Lisa. But again, it wasn't the same Fred," he recalled.

As it turned out, the two of them had been assigned seats next to each other. Lisa knew of Fred's health challenges and was delighted to hear his situation was improving. He had not been aware of the battle Lisa was facing.

"She said she was undergoing some cancer treatments," Fred recalled. "She said it in such a matter-of-fact way. I said, 'Lisa, I think so much of City of Hope. You need to go there for a second opinion.' That night she texted me. She said, 'I've talked to Chuck, and we're going to do this.'"

Fred was quickly in touch with his friend and City of Hope patient navigator Lupe Santana, who told Fred to have Lisa contact her. A few weeks after that, Lisa Bowman and her husband drove onto the City of Hope campus for the first time.

"I couldn't believe I was there because I always heard City of Hope was difficult to get into," she remembered. "They were just so wonderful. The valet parking guy said, 'Parking is free your first time here, and I just want you to know you're in the right place. We're going to take care of you.' This was the guy parking your car! I looked at Chuck, and he looked at me, and we kind of went, 'Wow.'"

As she settled into her treatment, Lisa began to hear the stories of people who had come to City of Hope after being told elsewhere that they had run out of medical options.

"Then they get to City of Hope, and someone there takes one look and says, 'We've seen this before, and here is what we're going to do,' and then they end up being okay," Lisa said.

But to her, the spirit of kindness at City of Hope was as healing as the medicine.

"I made a list of the things that I loved the most about the place," she said. "Of all the hospitals and places that I've been to, they had by far the most extensive collection of wigs and beauty products that can help a woman get through this, because you really do feel mutilated. It's tough. I had long hair. Right before my hair was going to fall out, the woman in the beauty shop said, 'Let me cut it short. It will make it easier when it falls out.' And it did. It really and truly did.

"There really is a basic human kindness to the place, a duality," she continued. "There is this incredible organization. But there are also gardens. They make the place beautiful, with the fountain and running water. That's really important to healing. Even though it's subtle, when you hear water running and you see beautiful colors and it's such a clean place, all of that is really subconsciously important."

Lisa felt it was the place she was meant to be.

"Fred wouldn't have gone there if it hadn't been a special place," she said in January 2020 when her treatments were done and her cancer was at bay. "I trusted that. When I got there, I discovered that he was right."

•◆•

Doctors eventually traced Fred Claire's latest medical issue to a bad tooth. In other circumstances, a tooth infection would have been a relatively minor thing, especially when compared to the litany of grave health challenges he had faced over the last three years at City of Hope. But the infection had spread to the section of jaw that had been compromised by the intensive radiation treatments of 2016. More specifically, the bone's vascular system had been damaged, and the resulting lack of blood flow made the jaw vulnerable to bacterial attack and less likely to heal once an infection had set in.

Fred's doctors were left with a menu of difficult treatment options. The most drastic was a sectional mandibulectomy, the same procedure that Gernon had proposed in 2016. But the delicate and invasive operation—cutting out the damaged section of his jaw and replacing it with a piece of bone taken from Fred's leg—had now become even riskier.

The surgery and rehabilitation would be grueling. Though in good health for a person his age, Fred Claire was three years older now, and his body had already been pushed to the limit. Surgeons would also have to negotiate dense scar tissue from the radiation treatments and, ultimately, any operation on weakened and compromised bone and tissue greatly increased the risk of complications.

"Because of the radiation, the skin overlying the soft tissue was almost like wood, it was so hard," said Dr. Sanjeet Dadwal, an oncologist and infectious disease specialist at City of Hope. "If you operate, there is a real concern about whether it will heal. And if it doesn't heal, you're left with bigger problems. He was not a good candidate for surgery."

That's why Fred's medical team undertook extreme measures to attempt to forestall the operation. Beginning April 10, 2019, at Gernon's recommendation, Claire underwent forty days of treatment in a hyperbaric oxygen chamber at Arcadia Methodist Hospital near City of Hope. During the ninety-minute sessions, known as dives, the air pressure inside the chamber was tripled, forcing more oxygen into Fred's lungs and thus into his bloodstream. More highly oxygenated blood had been shown effective in fighting infections and restoring bone and tissue damaged by radiation.

The supervising physician, Robert Cole, was a big baseball fan and had a Dodger jersey hung near Fred Claire's chamber for each dive, but the treatments had no discernible effect.

•◆•

When Fred and Sheryl Claire met Dadwal, he was about to celebrate fifteen years at City of Hope.

"It's been a nice journey, probably the best place to work," Dadwal said. "I do research. I do other stuff. But when it comes to patients, we all drop everything else. The patients come first."

Like so many of his colleagues, Dadwal had trained and worked in medical centers where doctors were constantly harried, competition was fierce, and the needs of patients often seemed secondary.

"At other places, you've got fifteen or twenty minutes to see a patient," Dadwal said. "Here, if you need to see a patient for forty minutes, you see them for forty minutes. You spend your time with a patient. That's how you develop relationships, develop trust. You can't do that in fifteen minutes. If patients don't feel safe and comfortable, what will their journey be like? Confused. Anxious. That's not what you want in a cancer hospital."

In the painful spring of 2019, Dadwal became an important member of Fred's medical team, and a close relationship quickly developed between doctor and patient. After the hyperbaric oxygen treatments, Dadwal attacked Fred's infection with daily intravenous infusions of powerful antibiotics.

"I'm a physician, and I have to know everything about a patient to make an impact," Dadwal said. "But Fred and Sheryl were also very nice. They asked about my family and how I balanced home life with the amount of time I work. That's how we came to discuss our kids. Fred has been a role model to many young people, helping to develop them, and he started asking about my older son, asked what he was doing."

Dadwal showed Fred and Sheryl a video from a recent family trip to their native India, filmed by the physician's sixteen-year-old son, Jay, who was an aspiring filmmaker. Fred told the doctor there was someone he wanted Jay to meet.

Michael Trim, a producer and director with a long list of movie and television credits, was part of Fred's breakfast group at Pie 'n Burger. One day at the Pasadena restaurant, Fred arranged for Trim to sit down with the cancer specialist and his teenage son.

"Fred went out of his way to introduce Jay to someone in the industry," Dadwal said. "During that breakfast, when my son stepped away from the table, Fred told me, 'I've met a lot of young people in my life. You don't have to worry about your son. He will be successful. At sixteen, he knows what he wants to do.' Fred is eighty-three years old. He had tons of experience. He ran the Dodgers for God knows how many years. And after one hour he was able to tell me, 'Dr. Dadwal, you don't have to worry about this boy.' It was really amazing."

But Fred's condition continued to deteriorate. When the problematic tooth was extracted in May, follow-up scans revealed a hairline fracture in the jaw. The compromised bone would never heal in its blood-deprived state, and high doses of antibiotics seemed only minimally effective in combating the infection. Fred was in constant pain and could not chew solid foods because of the instability in his jaw.

"It's not just that my bite would not be the same day to day. It would not be the same from bite to bite," Fred remembered.

His doctors noticed a change in their previously indomitable patient.

"He was miserable. I could just see it," Gernon recalled. "He wasn't talking. He was subdued. He just wasn't himself."

By July, the surgery the medical team had endeavored so mightily to avoid began to look more and more inevitable, though the patient remained hesitant.

"Fred said, 'Well, my life really isn't that bad,'" Gernon recalled. "I said, 'You're not really the same person you were when you came in here.' And I could tell Sheryl was stressed by it. So, we started talking about doing the original surgery. That was the best bet, to cut out the dead jawbone and bring in vascularized bone. It was risky because he had done this previous surgery in 2016 and had chemo and radiation, so there could be post-op issues."

Fred eventually decided to go ahead. "I didn't want to go on like that," he said. "There had to be a risk to get to a reward. This surgery has been done. These are the guys who can do it. But the bottom line is that there was no other practical option."

Fred received his last infusion of intravenous antibiotics on July 30. Before leaving City of Hope, he and his wife stopped by Gernon's office.

"Let's do it," Sheryl Claire said.

The surgery was scheduled for the following day.

• ◆ •

Gernon had performed the operation, a sectional mandibulectomy, on dozens of previous patients, but the compromised anatomy of Fred's neck and jaw would make this surgery one of the most challenging of his career.

"Any time you do that surgery with a patient that has already had chemo and radiation, the risk of complication goes way, way up," Gernon recalled. "We had a plan. I really thought it out, but it was hard. It was really hard."

He would be joined in the operating room by Dr. Robert Kang and Dr. Ellie Maghami. The boyish looking Kang, a rock guitarist and singer in a band called Help the Doctor, had been a close friend of Gernon's since they were both in surgical training at the University of Washington School of Medicine. Maghami was the head of City of Hope's head and neck surgical department and a leading national expert in the field. She had first met Gernon at Kang's Malibu wedding in 2016 and recruited Gernon after that.

"I could have searched the world and not found more comfort in the people who were going to be doing the surgery," Fred said.

Kang would be responsible for harvesting a section of Fred's fibula, a smaller, non-weight bearing bone in the patient's leg.

"That's what makes the surgery possible," Kang explained later. "You can remove it, but you can still walk and run without that bone."

After a tourniquet was applied to stop blood flow to the leg, Kang worked his way through the skin and soft tissue to reach the fibula, clamping off an artery and vein leading into the bone before removing the bone itself. Then the surgical team was on the clock. The piece of fibula would die within six hours if blood flow was not restored.

"There is no oxygen or blood going into it," Kang explained. "Once you clip this artery and vein, the bone is holding its breath."

Working on the patient's neck, Gernon found the scar tissue denser and more problematic than he had anticipated. In that difficult environment, the surgeon needed to locate a healthy vein and artery that could be mated to vessels from the transplanted fibula.

"There was a lot of fibrosis scar tissue," Gernon said. "We had to get through all of that, digging new blood vessels out of all this scar. Finding good blood vessels is difficult, and you have to establish good blood flow through those vessels, or the transplanted bone will die. You're at risk of losing the whole reconstruction, having to throw it in the garbage, and start over because the blood isn't flowing through the bone."

As he worked, Gernon grappled with another concern—that he might come across previously undetected tumors.

"Cancer usually falls apart when you're in it," Gernon said. "It's a cheesy material. I kept sending specimen after specimen to the pathology lab to look at this white, fibrous tissue. I kept taking this stuff out, and they kept telling me it was just scar. They never found any evidence of cancer."

Hours into the surgery, Gernon managed to locate and tease out the necessary vein and artery. He was stunned when he got to the jawbone itself. It had virtually disintegrated, meaning that the surgery, as difficult as it was, had truly been Fred's only hope. When the bone was cut out, Gernon laid the piece of fibula in a titanium plate molded to the contour of Fred's jaw. Then he and Kang began connecting the delicate plumbing.

"Under a microscope, using sutures the size of a hair, you sew artery to artery and vein to vein," Kang said "You're still on the clock. When that's done and everything looks like it's connected, you take off the clamps. You breathe a sigh of relief when the blood with the oxygen flows through the bone and the deoxygenated blood flows out through the vein. You watch it for a while to make sure it looks alive. Then you have your reconstruction."

• ◆ •

Fred was eighty-three years old on the day of the grueling, eight-hour surgery.

"I asked T.J. more than once, even on the day before in his office, 'You're sure he's going to get through this?'" Sheryl said. "He didn't seem to have any doubt, but you never know."

She spent the day of the surgery in a waiting room with Lupe Santana and friend Rich Kee, receiving periodic updates from nurses, making detailed notes and keeping Fred's daughters, Jennifer and Kim, and her own friends and family informed about the surgery's progress.

"She was obviously very anxious—very positive, but she wanted as much detail as possible," Kee recalled. "That's her guy, and it was a very unnerving time. But that day wasn't any different from the way she handled herself on day one at City of Hope. She's very thorough. She wants to be as informed as possible. She wants to be sure nothing falls through the cracks. That's not a dig at any of the medical staff, but she's there because she was his best advocate."

It was late in the afternoon that Gernon and Kang finally walked through the door of the waiting room in their scrubs. Sheryl was relieved the moment she saw them.

"They had been in surgery for eight hours, and they walked in looking like they were ready to pose for GQ magazine," she remembered. "It was unbelievable. They said everything went fine. Mission accomplished. I was just relieved to know that it was over."

But her heart sank when she entered the recovery room. The left side of her husband's face had ballooned to twice its normal size. Though awake, Fred Claire was attached to breathing and feeding tubes and could not speak.

"I went to the side of his bed, held his hand, touched his arm, and kissed him on his forehead," Sheryl said. "It was difficult to look at the size of his face, and he looked stunned. After the first surgery in 2016, he was talking right away. With this one there were no words. I told him I loved him, and he just nodded. It was just a very, very long surgery."

The next morning, she watched as two physical therapists and a nurse attempted to get Fred out of bed.

"He's lying in bed, and his face is swollen like a pumpkin," Sheryl said. "It took them fifteen to twenty minutes to get Fred sitting up on the side of the bed with all the wires and tubes hanging from him. They got him up with a belt around his waist, and they had him take two little steps to the left and that was it. That was when I thought to myself, 'This is going to be a very long recovery.'"

But by the next day, Fred was up and making his way around his room. When driving back to City of Hope a few days after the surgery, Sheryl received a phone call from a familiar number.

"I thought, 'How can it be Fred calling? He's still got a breathing tube and can't talk.'" she remembered. "I pulled over to the side of the road and called him back. He said, 'How do you like my new voice?' And on one of the first days after surgery, he sent me a selfie and was smiling."

In those early days, a steady stream of familiar faces stopped by to check on Fred, among them City of Hope doctors Stephen Forman, Steven Rosen, and Sanjeet Dadwal.

"I went to see him the second day he was out of surgery," Dadwal said. "He still couldn't talk, so he wrote on a piece of paper, 'How is Jay doing? How is his project coming along?' I said, 'You rest. You don't have to worry about that right now. I'll let you know.'"

A few days after the surgery, when Fred had his cell phone back, Rich Kee sent him a text message that said how proud of him everyone was.

Kee said, "Here's his reply: 'Rich, we all get tested. Who we are is determined by how we handle the challenges.' I mean it stopped me in my tracks. This sums up his entire journey. He was in a bed and had just had half of his jaw removed, and he's got a fight and uncertainty ahead, and he comes up with something like that. That's why we all admire him."

Dr. Massarelli came by Fred's room with the best news of all.

"My personal victory was when they took the jaw out and cut it into little slices and analyzed it in the pathology lab," Fred's oncologist remembered later. "There was no cancer. I thought, 'My gosh. We have won. We know that there is no cancer there. The immune system has really been able to kill the cancer. Oh my God.' It really was like a miracle to me."

Soon, Fred was making laps around the hospital floor with the help of a walker, hauling an IV pole with him.

"We were walking around the floor of the hospital one day, and I said, 'Fred, you just need to take steps. You don't need to race or break any records,'" Sheryl recalled. "And the physical therapist turned to me and said, 'I think he just did.' It was miraculous."

Thirteen days after the surgery, Fred was discharged from City of Hope. He and his wife returned to their home in Pasadena, where a basketball hoop hangs in the driveway and neighbors occasionally see two senior citizens shooting baskets.

"The days were longer in summer, and I could walk and nap and get up and walk again," Fred remembered in January 2020. "I was determined to do the exercises, and I knew I had to strengthen my neck and heal the wound in my leg. But I never viewed it as a finish line. I've never viewed it as having won the race. I really viewed it, and continue to view it, as a marathon. The key part for me is to find joy in the running of the marathon. Even today, that's really the key. You have to find joy in each and every day, no matter the challenges you may face."

• ◆ •

One afternoon in October 2019, at the end of another long day at City of Hope, Gernon sat in his office, reflecting on the remarkable journey of the patient who had become a friend.

Gernon said, "Even though it wasn't a known cancer diagnosis, he had to relive all those same emotions with the jaw surgery and know we were doing it in a high-risk setting. But it went well, and he got through it and is doing great. From the medical perspective, it's been something, but Fred to me now is much more than a patient."

Gernon said he occasionally exchanged text messages with Fred on difficult days.

"This is a tough job sometimes, and he helps me reset," Gernon said.

The surgeon recalled quiet moments in Fred's room after the operation, talking about things other than the challenging case.

"I would sit in his room and talk about life," Gernon said. "He just has so much wisdom. I remember I was watching a baseball game with him, and he said, 'You know, that guy is making twenty-five million a year. Who needs that much money to do that sport?' He's just refreshing. He's down-to-Earth. He's centered for the common good. There is so much to learn from him. He's just a person for others."

That afternoon during the interview, Gernon described a phone conversation he had with Fred a few days before: "I could hear the wind, so I said, 'You're on the golf course, aren't you? He's like, 'I'm hitting balls with Sheryl.' That's more like Fred to me."

•◆•

On November 5, 2019, the best of Dodger blue once again gathered to support one of their own. The occasion was the annual Ross Porter Celebrity Golf Classic benefitting Stillpoint Family Resources, a nonprofit organization that assists adults with special needs.

Forty-two years earlier, Fred Claire had helped hire Porter, then a local sports anchorman, to join Vin Scully in the Dodger broadcast booth. By the time of his departure in 2004, Porter was one of the most beloved media personalities in franchise history. That autumn day at El Caballero Country Club in Tarzana, Scully was among those in attendance, joining Tommy Lasorda, Mike Scioscia, Mickey Hatcher, and—just three months after his agonizing surgery—Fred Claire.

It was not lost on the former general manager that this latest reunion took place on the fiftieth anniversary of his joining the Dodgers. For Fred and Sheryl, who also attended Porter's tournament, the meaning of the day was greatly magnified by what they had just endured.

"Here we were with Ross, whom I had a hand in bringing to the Dodgers as an announcer," Fred recalled. "He has remained a great friend. His tournament was an inspiration for my own, and Ross was so generous to emcee both of them. And here we were with Tommy and Vin. There aren't two more iconic names in the last fifty years of Dodger history than those two. They were both in their nineties, I was in my eighties, and Sheryl and I had just been through it all. To have another chance to experience their friendship and warmth and touch all that history, it doesn't get any better than that."

As was so often the case over the years, Rich Kee was on hand that day to capture special moments with his camera. Lasorda had yet to arrive at Porter's tournament when the photographer gathered five longtime friends for a portrait. In the picture, Scully is seated. Standing behind him are Ron Roenicke (who came up with the Dodgers as a young player, later managed the Milwaukee Brewers and is the current manager of the Boston Red Sox), Mike Scioscia, Fred Claire, and Mickey Hatcher. Roenicke, Claire, and Hatcher each rest a hand on Scully's shoulder, and the five of them are smiling with great delight at something one of them has said.

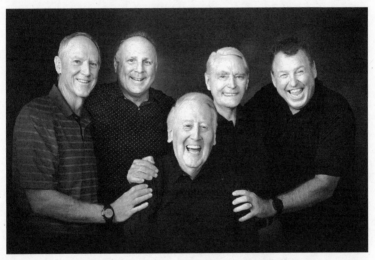

Vin Scully is front and center as friends and former Dodgers (from left) Ron Roenicke, Mike Scioscia, Fred, and Mickey Hatcher gather at Ross Porter's celebrity golf tournament in 2019.

The resulting photograph would be among the most evocative of Kee's long career.

"When I showed it to Fred, his reaction was, 'Rich, just look at this. This goes to show the love we have for Vin,'" Kee recalled.

"But the more I looked at it, the more I realized how much it showed the love those five guys had for each other."

Claire would later put it more simply.

"What that picture says to me is this," he said. "We are Dodgers."

•◆•

That year's holiday season was the most painless and anxiety-free that Fred and Sheryl Claire had spent in recent years. There were still regular trips to City of Hope for physical therapy and occupational therapy, an occasional scan, and other follow-up appointments, but more and more they resumed what resembled a normal life. Hours sometimes passed without either of them thinking about their remarkable journey of healing.

But from time to time it would all come back: The moments of terror, exhaustion, and despair that were always followed by gestures of compassion, love, and hope. In their memories was a kaleidoscope of faces from City of Hope, from the world's most renowned physicians and researchers, to the nurses and therapists, as well as people they knew only by their first names and their smiles—the young man at the entrance check-in desk, the clerks in the pharmacy, the baristas at the City of Hope Starbucks. Each felt like family now.

They would think of departed friends, like Kevin Towers, Tom Quinley, and the young employee at City of Hope who worked on Fred's first golf tournament and later lost her battle with ovarian cancer. Not a day would go by without some reminder that Fred Claire was the only one of four patients to survive the same clinical trial. Tears crept into Sheryl Claire's eyes whenever she thought of the families of the other patients.

The Claires pondered all they had been through with a sense of wonder and gratitude. Each day, each hour became even more of a gift. Fred Claire would say, quite simply, he was "blessed."

At Ross Porter's golf tournament, Rich Kee took another deeply meaningful photograph, this one of Fred and Sheryl. In it, she rests her hands on her husband's shoulders. After years of heartache and worry, her smile conveys a deep peace. Fred Claire beams at the camera, the scars of his recent surgery barely noticeable.

The Claires chose Kee's photograph as their holiday greeting card for 2019, a card that also bore a one-word message:

"Joy."

ACKNOWLEDGMENTS

Those three days in the spring of 2019, my introduction to City of Hope, were among the most profound of my career as a writer and journalist. They began with a late-afternoon interview with CEO Robert Stone, who was clearly weary, but warmed immediately to our topic, the combination of cutting-edge science and compassion that has made his institution unique in the annals of American medicine.

"There is a humility to people here who recognize that what we can do together is profoundly more impactful than what anyone can do alone," Stone said. "If you really put people at the center, you see how we can help cancer patients and their families across the world."

Then, the next day, in a conference room at City of Hope, I sat down with some of the world's most renowned clinicians and researchers, Stephen Forman, Steven Rosen, Joseph Alvarnas, T.J. Gernon, and Erminia Massarelli. We discussed recent breakthroughs in cancer treatment, particularly as they applied to the case of Fred Claire.

But what I will always remember most was how much each of them reminded me of another friend of mine, Fred Rogers, the icon of children's television. I had met *that* Fred in 1995 through a newspaper assignment and remained close to him until his death eight years later. I was thus able to witness first-hand true, human greatness—his deep presence, profound compassion, kindness, and wisdom.

I recognized those same qualities in the people I met at City of Hope and, as a result, came away believing that the place is a model not just for medicine, but for humanity more generally, especially at this difficult moment in history.

It was my great fortune to meet many others on that first trip to City of Hope, in a subsequent visit, or in telephone conversations during the research for this book. They include Arthur Riggs, Ellie Maghami, Badri Modi, Sanjeet Dadwal, Robert Kang, Saul Priceman, Ashley Baker Lee, Mahjabeen Hashmi, and Lupe Santana. My thanks to them all, and to my friend, Josh Jenisch, and his amazing staff, who worked tirelessly to facilitate my work at the medical center.

My first real acquaintance with the Los Angeles Dodgers came when I was six years old, pulling against the Dodgers as they faced my beloved Minnesota Twins in the 1965 World Series. Alas, the Dodgers won in seven games. Despite that early disappointment, I've been a serious baseball fan ever since. I remember marveling at Orel Hershiser's historic mastery in 1988 and was watching on television when Kirk Gibson hit his historic home run. Which is a very long way of saying how much fun it was for me to visit with former major league players, broadcasters, and executives who are part of the Fred Claire story.

I'm particularly grateful to Peter O'Malley for his insight and candor in our two interviews. I greatly enjoyed two long and highly entertaining conversations with Kirk Gibson, and another with Rick Dempsey. My thanks also to Vin Scully, Tommy Lasorda, Mike Scioscia, Joey Amalfitano, John Shelby,

Mickey Hatcher, Peter Bavasi, Phil Regan, Sandy Alderson, and Tim Belcher.

The story of Kevin Towers, his courageous and inspiring battle with cancer and his friendship with Fred, is such an important part of this story, and I'm indebted to those who helped me tell it. My thanks to Barry Axelrod and Bob Nightengale, but particularly to Kelley Towers. Kevin's spirit and memory live on in so many ways.

The story of Tom Quinley, Jaylon Fong, and South Hills High School baseball seems worthy of a book (and a movie) in itself. Thanks to Bill Quinley, John Sherrard, Chris Woodward, Darren Murphy, Jaylon's father, Francis Fong, and Jaylon himself.

It has been my great pleasure and privilege to get to know so many of the fine people who are part of Fred and Sheryl's world. The great *Los Angeles Times* writer Bill Plaschke is one of them. We are humbled by the words in his foreword to this book. Our gratitude to Dodger manager Dave Roberts for his friendship to Fred and his support for *Extra Innings*.

I'm grateful to Lisa Bowman, who so generously shared her own experience at City of Hope. My thanks also to Ann Meyers Drysdale, Ben Hwang, Ari Kaplan, Jeff Fellenzer, and Merri Ann Irons.

Rich Kee deserves special mention here. No person could be a more devoted friend than Rich is to Fred and Sheryl. I also benefitted greatly by the fact that Rich was present at so many of the important moments in this story and described them for me with a poet's heart and a writer's eye for detail. I'm very happy to call Rich my friend.

Kudos to Naren Aryal, Nicole Hall, and the team at Mascot Books.

All of my books are dedicated to my wife, Catherine, our children, Melanie and Patrick, and now, Patrick's fiancée, Alison. In this time of pandemic, it's only fitting to give a nod to the family dogs, Scuba and Gordo, who have given us such unconditional love and much-needed distraction in these difficult times.

Which brings me to Fred and Sheryl. I mentioned earlier my friendship with Fred Rogers, a historically great human being. In my mind, the Claires fall into that category themselves. Both Claires are unfailingly kind, thoughtful, and funny (especially Sheryl). But there is a quiet intensity to them both, a fierce commitment to doing what is right and serving others, no matter what the circumstances, however difficult they might be. In that they have much in common with the people at City of Hope.

Fred Rogers once said something to the effect that one of life's greatest challenges is to make goodness attractive. That has not been a problem here. This is a story for our time. It has been my privilege to help tell it.

Tim Madigan